You Have Ovarian Cancer
"Four Words That Changed Our Lives Forever"

**Stories by Women/Girls Afflicted with
Ovarian Cancer and their Loved Ones**

3G Publishing, Inc.
Loganville, Ga 30052
www.3gpublishinginc.com
Phone: 1-888-442-9637

First published by 3G Publishing, Inc. November, 2016

ISBN: 9781941247365

Printed in the United States of America

Contents

Foreword   *9*

Introduction   *15*

Chapter 1   *17*
HOPE
Between Home and Oz

Chapter 2   *21*
Why Does My Baby Have Ovarian
    Cancer?

Chapter 3   *27*
"What Will You Tell the Children?"

Chapter 4   *33*
What Are We Going to Do?

Chapter 5   *37*
The Journey

Chapter 6   *43*
The Cruelness of Ovarian Cancer

Chapter 7   *59*
Our Story

Chapter 8   *63*
The Unimaginable—My Little Girl
  has Ovarian Cancer

Chapter 9   *67*
Through Ovarian Cancer
  I Built a Solid Foundation
  with God

Chapter 10   *85*
My Fifteen Year Battle
  with Ovarian Cancer

Chapter 11   *91*
Mom is Here to Stay

Chapter 12   *99*
Courage I Never Knew I Had

Chapter 13   *105*
Ana's Angels Teal the End

Chapter 14   *109*
Lunch & Learn Saved my Life

Chapter 15   *119*
"This is the Day the Lord has made,
   I will rejoice and be glad in it!"
Psalms 118:24

Chapter 16   *143*
God's Handiwork

Chapter 17   *155*
My Intent for the Remainder of
   My LIFE

Chapter 18   *167*
Prayer Availeth Much

Chapter 19   *169*
Self-Diagnosing

Chapter 20   *177*
In the Best Shape of my LIFE

Chapter 21   *187*
Hope is Passion for What is Possible
   "Live, Laugh and Love"

Chapter 22   *193*
God Does Have a Plan

Chapter 23   *197*
Love Had Nothing to Do With It

Chapter 24   *203*
Not a Way to Bring in The New Year

Chapter 25   *209*
Ovarian Cancer Through the
   Eyes of a Son

Chapter 26   *215*
It's a Whole New World

Chapter 27   *223*
I Am to Young to Have
   Ovarian Cancer

Chapter 28   *231*
Love at First Sight

Chapter 29   *237*
I Believe In Miracles

Chapter 30   *261*
**Blank Stares, Salt Shakers, Robots
  and a Better Me**

Foreword

Denise Wyllie and I met in London where we live, in the Spring of 2001. Being confident women artists, we began working together almost immediately sharing skills and resources.

Denise, generous by nature, invited me to join her in an art / science residency at a Cancer Research UK funded laboratory in London.

We worked for two years at University College London Hospital and made a monumental 42 metre cross media textile artwork, "Transformations in Science and Art". This artwork celebrates the growing awareness of the importance of DNA in Cancer Research, and the positive developments in drug therapies over the last 50 years. A large format digital print of this is in permanent exhibition at The Royal Mint Building, by Tower Bridge in London.

In tandem to this work, we wanted to help people whose lives have been affected by cancer. We ran a series of workshops where people made a small textile artwork in white. Everybody had their own story and reason to create an individual piece of whitework. Based on the outcomes created during the workshops we have just published a book called "Whitework – A Gentle Path. This shows the artworks and thoughts of those who took part and demonstrates that by focusing on creative therapy a person can get some respite from the chaotic world that cancer brings. We are delighted to give 250 copies of this book for inclusion into GOCA's 'Bag of Hope" this year.

During our Art/Science Residency we discovered that the scientist

Rosalind Franklin made the first clear X-Ray image of the structure of DNA while working at King's College in London in 1952. Franklin's photo Photo 51 led to the discovery of the double helix by James Watson and Francis Crick for which they received a Nobel Prize. Her work was used without permission or acknowledgement at the time and Photo 51 proved to be a driving force behind one of the greatest discoveries in the history of science. We made a series of contemporary art prints called "The Rosalind Franklin Collection" where we celebrate her achievements. Rosalind Franklin died at the age of 37 from ovarian cancer.

The shock of learning about Franklin's death had a profound effect on me. I was diagnosed with ovarian cancer shortly after meeting Denise. I was angry and believed that the lack of awareness of ovarian cancer amongst women, mirrored the lack of awareness we have on women's achievements in science and the workplace. Channeling the energy anger arises, we decided to put this to use to raise awareness of Franklin's work, and raise awareness of ovarian cancer at the same time.

I had hooked up with a network of ovarian cancer survivor activists online in the early 2000's and through that learned about the work of OCNA – The Ovarian Cancer National Alliance in Washington DC. Their work greatly impressed us: lobbying congress, holding conferences where medical experts shared information, implementing innovative expert patient programs etc. Through establishing a relationship with the organization Denise and I were invited to present our art work at OCNA's 8th Annual Conference in Atlanta. In addition to our presentation at the Conference, one of our artworks "A Vision of Rosalind I' was presented to Barbara Goff, MD for the inaugural 2005 Rosalind Franklin Excellence in Ovarian Cancer Research Award.

In Atlanta we met many fine women activists/advocates at the 2005 conference, including Ginger Ackerman (deceased) - President of

OCNA and Founder Member of GOCA; Janet Rigdon, (deceased) – Director South Carolina Ovarian Cancer Foundation, Greenville. We agreed to work with them, using our art to support awareness raising missions of ovarian cancer. Members and supporters of the ovarian cancer community deliver on their promises - if you say you are going to do something, you do it – it's not simply a vague intention.

Just the evening before we arrived in Atlanta, Denise and I attended an Art Auction, called "Love Art", at Coutts Bank in The Strand, London. In May 2005, we were commissioned to make a series of four original art prints for this event by Ovarian Cancer Action, a UK organization which supports scientific research and awareness raising missions. We named our new series of art prints "The Hope that Surrounds Us' and since 2007, the four images together form the logo for GOCA.

In approaching the commission for Ovarian Cancer Action, Denise and I considered how we could describe a different view of the experience of cancer, both visually and in words. When diagnosed with ovarian cancer, I struggled to find roles models that would suit me. In 2005, cyclist, cancer survivor and activist Lance Armstrong won his seventh Tour de France. Reading press coverage at that time, I reacted really strongly against the competitive, combative model of cancer survivorship he embodied. To me, the language of cancer is and continues to be very limiting. I remembered being exhausted by people urging me to be positive. At a time of experiencing great pain and a great fear of dying I found great relief when the word "hope' entered my vocabulary. One could have more flexibility with "hope' – a little hope, a faint hope, hope, some hope, lots of hope and great hope as opposed to positive and negative which offers no movement at all.

Ovarian cancer resides in a place in our bodies where a life begins. Those of us who face ovarian cancer, are aware that it may be the place where the end of our life begins. What we need is hope – hope that we will be able to manage a way through an uncertain future with some peace.

We made the idea of hope central to the new artworks. In preparing to write the foreword to this book, we researched our archive and found the original aims for the art prints. In 2005 we wrote; "to look at the work as an act of affirmation – a mantra – a prayer – in engaging with the work we allow ourselves time to experience a Moments peace knowing that hope surrounds us – have a vision of cancer that contains hope and beauty."

The artwork 'The Hope that Surrounds Us, is a creative visual response to the the limitations imposed by words when describing the experience of cancer. Visual imagery is the most direct and powerful way to communicate meaning. To make the work we began by making a study of biological drawings of the ovary. The shape of the ovary suggested an enclosed space and our intention was to amplify this to make a safe place, where we will be held in its embrace. People often ask us how do we work together? In this instance, I made the drawings whilst Denise worked on creating calm complimentary colours.

We discussed ways in which "The Hope that Surrounds Us' could be used to further ovarian cancer awareness with Janet Rigdon in Atlanta in 2005. Following on from our resolve to work together, the artwork was central to a South Carolina Ovarian Cancer Foundation exhibition event in 2006, in Greenville. An exhibition of our work on Rosalind Franklin was also shown in Charleston in 2007 at the Smith Killian Fine Art Gallery hosted by Jennet Alterman at The Center for Women.

Janet Rigdon worked closely with GOGA and through her I met Marjorie Rosing who made the request to use our art prints as GOCA's logo. We knew about the work of GOCA through Ginger

Ackerman and in February 2007, we signed off on that.

We are so delighted to see that our "hope", our "strong and confident expectations" for our art have been surpassed with GOCA. They have embraced it and made it work. When making the original work, in our studio in London, we never imagined our "The Hope that Surrounds Us" would be emblazoned on a racing car driving on the US Indy circuit, or on a boat in tournament fishing. These innovative, creative approaches reaches new audiences in awareness raising missions. We salute GOCA and hope that their aims are realized in increased awareness and education of women, their families, as well as the health care community about risks, symptoms, and treatment of ovarian cancer leading to earlier detection.

Clare O Hagan and Denise Wyllie
http://www.wyllieohagan.com
email: info@wyllieohagan.com

About Wyllie O Hagan

Wyllie O Hagan: Denise Wyllie and Clare O Hagan are visual artists. activists and filmmakers, living in London. Together, the two artists tackle and deliver huge art projects and exhibitions. These are ambitious in scale and concept conveying complex aspects of the human condition. With their wide professional experience, they utilize a range of media within their moving image film work, using paintings, prints, textiles and land art.

The scale of their works range from small works on paper to a monumental transient land print the size of a football pitch. One project "Transformations in Science and Art", a 42 metre cross media work is on permanent exhibition in the Royal Mint Building, London.

Wyllie O Hagan recent moving image artworks have appeared both in gallery exhibition and screened at film festivals internationally. This work is held in The Archive of Film, New

York and The Australian Centre for Moving Image, Melbourne Australia, and The Karelian State Museum Collection, Russia.

Images, with information in the titles sent separately.
Please ask for further information on captioning images if required.

Introduction

"You have ovarian cancer." These four words are heard by approximately 22,000 women and their families every year.

Anybody can find and recite the risks and symptoms of ovarian cancer as well as memorize and quote statistics. However, only a few can truly tell you what those four words really mean.

These are their stories. They provide a glimpse of how those four words have impacted their lives.

You will read first person ovarian cancer experiences comprising of love, fear, hope, pain, strength, loss, courage, faith, perseverance, luck and every emotion possible.

Each story is unique of itself but one common thing is evident, ovarian cancer does not discriminate.

Doug Barron, Executive Director

Chapter 1

HOPE
Between Home and Oz

By Larry & Donna Aber
(Parents of Rachel Marie Aber)

December 18, 2005, Rachel Marie Aber graduated from The University of Georgia and I was as proud as a daddy could be. The night before, I wrote her a letter. It went with her graduation gift from her Mom, Donna and I, a three stone diamond necklace. It was a very happy day.

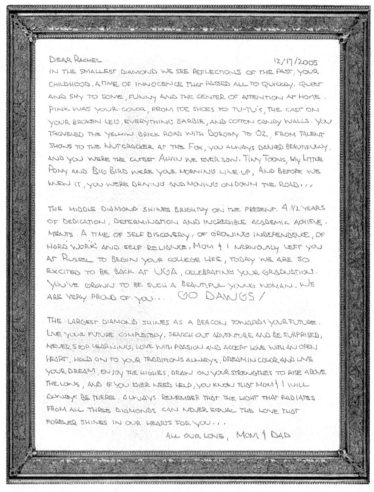

"[16] For God so loved the world that he gave his one and only Son, that whoever believes in him shall not perish but have eternal life."
John 3:16 (NIV)

August 30, 2007, it was a sunny day outside, our pager beeped and we hurried to catch the elevator to the surgical waiting room floor. The doors opened and Rachel's doctor was standing there. That's when Rachel's Mom and I heard the words, "Rachel's mass is malignant, and it is ovarian cancer." Everything for me went gray, and I knew our lives were about to be changed forever.

This was not supposed to happen, it was not part of our plan. Rachel was to turn 25 years old in October, she was engaged just one week earlier, worked out daily, ate fish and broccoli, was a proud Georgia Bulldog, had a fantastic job and bright future, wonderful friends to grow old with, and a proud, loving and supporting family.

After a long day and late night, Rachel was finally settled in her soon to be, all too familiar hospital room. Mom of course, spending the night by her bedside. Rachel told her Mom she needed a word to get her through the fight that she already seemed to know lay ahead. Rachel chose the HOPE.

HOPE: To cherish a desire with expectation of obtainment.

After Rachel's passing, HOPE become our word to the battle cry for Team Rachel's HOPE, started by her childhood friend Heather. An army of friends, friends of friends, and family, a legacy in memory of Rachel to fight the fight for all who are touched by ovarian cancer.

INSPIRE: To excite, encourage and breathe life into others.

Rachel wanted to be an inspiration to others. Her work ethic and dedication to her employer Trimont was truly amazing, chemo nurses, doctors, and other patients were her second family, and her self-made video of HOPE, FAITH, and FAMILY continues to inspire others worldwide on Rachelshope.net, a website dedicated to ovarian cancer, created by her Uncle Ken and Aunt Carol. During her 14 month battle filled with chemo and test, hospital stays too

19

numerous to remember, the seemingly always present pain, Rachel fought her fight with strength and grace. She lived her life to the fullest. She laughed and cried with friends, supported others in their time of need, did her fair share of what she called "Retail Therapy", and brought a sense of HOPE and PEACE, to her Mom, her big brother Derek and me.

OZ: The land where gray turns into the colors of the rainbow.

October 20, 2008 we know Rachel finally reached her OZ, because she was home where she wanted to be. Her Mom, her brother and I held her hands, softly kissed her as she peacefully passed from this life to the next. And then our angel smiled her beautiful smile, a memory that will live in our hearts forever and always.

November 26, 2008 at 2:38pm, we placed Rachel's ashes into the warm water of the Gulf of Mexico. Her Uncle Chuck and Aunt Laurie charted two beautiful sailboats, friends and family sailed on a brisk wind, taking Rachel to a spot just off the beach where she played as a little girl, where she could reach her destiny, to merge with infinity. The waters surface twinkled with sunlight and was laced with the colorful flotilla of handpicked flowers and rose petals. As we reached the dock and disembarked, Grandma Janson looked back over the tall swaying mast and said, "Look at the rainbow", the sky was the brightest blue, the cloud a wispy white, and in the center a square block of a rainbow called a Sea Dog by sailors. Rachel blessed us that day, as she continues to do from time to time. Rainbows appear, we feel her hug, we smile, and sometimes we cry, but we know she is blowing us a kiss and saying that everything will be alright.

I Love You Rachel

Rachel's Daddy, Larry

Chapter 2

Why Does My Baby Have Ovarian Cancer?

By Tammi Arrowood
(Mother of Audrey Arrowood)

On July 12, 2010, Audrey was placed on the fast track in Scottish Rite Children's Hospital's emergency department after an x-ray at our pediatrician's office revealed a mass in Audrey's abdomen. I was shocked that what I thought was constipation gave us such swift service. We'd hardly been inside the hospital ER when the nurse said, "The doctor's on his way down the hall". In fact, my husband was still parking the car as the nurse uttered those words. At that Moment, I knew we weren't dealing with constipation, and my heart fell to the floor. It was a whirlwind of activity. The doctor wanted an IV, CT scan, contrast and much more. None of us knew what was going on. After the CT scan, the ER doctor told us he wanted the Oncologist to see our daughter. I'm fairly certain the world stopped spinning on its axis for a few Moments because all I could think was, daughter and oncologist should NEVER be in the same sentence.

After speaking with the doctor, the nurses and the doctor wheeled Audrey around to the Aflac Cancer wing of Scottish Rite. I remember passing the sign that said "Aflac Cancer Center and Blood Disorders", feeling like I was having an out of body experience. The ER doctor must have noticed the look on my face because he said to me, "its okay, this is the best place for her right now," and he tugged on my elbow.

The CT scan revealed an "abnormal mass" was attached to her right ovary. Fortunately, most ovarian masses in children are benign. We stayed in our hospital room for 4 days until her surgery to remove the tumor. I held her in my arms and cried for her, and she never realized I shed a tear. Even though everyone was confident the mass was benign, I still couldn't wrap my mind around what was happening to our sweet, baby girl.

On July 16, 2010 the bombshell dropped. Dr. Woods and his PA came into our room while Audrey was recovering from surgery. They brought their own chairs and asked if we all could talk. At that point, my heart sank. He said the preliminary pathology results came in and Audrey does indeed have cancer, Ovarian Germ Cell Tumor. In fact, Dr. Woods revealed that Dr. Glasson, Audrey's surgeon, had removed a 3 lb. tumor, nearly the size of a basketball, from her right ovary. I just couldn't fathom that my 49 lb. daughter had been carrying something that big in her stomach. I looked over at my precious baby and wondered why and how. Again, the world, my world at least, stopped spinning on its axis but for far longer than a few Moments. Ironically, my mother had passed away from cancer 18 months before. Today's date, July 16, was my Mom's birthday. Surreal is the only word that came to mind.

The next day we met with Audrey's two oncologists. They walked us through the details of the next few months of our lives and immediately started making plans for chemotherapy, port placement and numerous medications. Mine and my husband's head spun as we had to take in the details of the ordeal our daughter would endure. We were initially told Audrey would only need four rounds of chemo. Those rounds would all be in-patient at the children's hospital.

All four rounds were completed in October. Audrey had another CT scan after completion, which revealed that her cancer had originally spread to her lymph nodes. Her original tumor was so large that it obscured the view of the cancerous lymph nodes. She immediately had a biopsy and confirmed her cancer had spread to her lymph nodes. They were removed and we prepared for two more rounds of chemo. We had already had our "celebration of completing chemo" before we found out about the cancerous lymph nodes. Once Audrey learned about the additional treatments, she was devastated. On the morning we had to leave for the first of her two more weeks of chemo, Audrey was nowhere to be found. We searched and searched and finally found her in our master closet behind hanging clothes and covered in piles of clothing. She begged us not to take her back. With tears streaming down her face, we picked her up kicking and screaming and wailing and buckled her into the car. We all felt so defeated. How could we do this to our precious baby, but then again, how could we not?

I never realized how much children with cancer have to endure. Audrey was constantly getting her port accessed, blood drawn, and antibiotics along with things like blood transfusions and vomiting and hair loss. My sweet, spunky girl would lay nearly lifeless in her hospital room fearing one tiny movement would cause her to vomit. My precious baby had never vomited in her life until chemo, and now she was vomiting up to 8 times an hour day after day. She'd go without food or drink for days, every smell or sight giving her dry heaves. The worst part to witness was upon completing her additional rounds of chemotherapy. Audrey stated having frequent panic attacks. We lived near the airport, and planes frequently flew over our house; they had for years. But now it was different. Every time Audrey was outside playing and a plane would fly overhead, she would run inside scream, cry, and hide in a corner yelling, "The plane is going to fall from the sky and kill me because cancer didn't!"

Another occasion occurred at a fast food restaurant. She begged me to take her home soon after arriving because she was terrified a robber would come in and kill her because cancer didn't. There were many different types of scenarios, but they all had this in common: "something is going to kill me because cancer didn't." The aftermath that cancer had on our family affected us all deeply. It especially effected Audrey's older brother.

Sadly, Audrey and I attended three funerals in the first eight months of her diagnosis. They were friends she made while in treatment. These 3 friends went through every available treatment, but it wasn't enough. Their cure couldn't be found. Prior to 1979, before the discovery of combination chemotherapy, only 27% of patients with stage I Ovarian Germ Cell (Endodermal Sinus) Tumor were alive at 2 years. Over 50% died within a year of diagnosis." Audrey's was a Stage 3 Ovarian Germ Cell (Endodermal Sinus) Tumor. If it weren't for research, my precious daughter wouldn't be here today. Fortunately, past cancer research saved her life!

We were so excited on her five year diagnosis anniversary! The end of scans. The end of blood draws. The end of oncology. Unfortunately, that celebration turned into unbearable fear yet again. Of all days, on her 5 year diagnosis anniversary and final scan, a new mass was found where her previous tumor had been 5 years earlier. That finding led to another lengthy surgery and my 13 year old started her seventh grade year in a wheelchair. We are so incredibly thankful the mass was benign, but that finding has led to MRI's every four months. So it seems, just when we thought our oncology days were coming to an end, here we are restarting the process with no end in sight to our oncology visits.

It has now been six years since her diagnosis, and we're thankful to announce she continues to remain cancer free! Albeit, the cancer monster has left scars in its path, scars that will be dealt with for the remainder of her life. She is at a higher risk to develop a secondary cancer due to her Etoposide treatment, and Audrey has hearing loss from the Cisplatin chemotherapy. The effects of her treatment will last a lifetime, although I praise God she's here to face these effects. So much more research is needed, for the fighters and for the survivors! The fighters deserve a chance at life, and the survivors deserve a chance not fraught with ongoing medical problems.

Chapter 3

"What Will You Tell the Children?"

By Heidi Barron
(Daughter of Wendy Sheron)

She was a healthy, happy 55 year old "Nana" to 5 grandchildren, living in Atlanta. Then everything changed when she went for her annual mammogram and was diagnosed with stage 1, ductal breast cancer on her grandson's second birthday. The diagnosis was sadly made immediately following her mother's death.

After a successful lumpectomy and radiation treatment, Wendy Sheron continued living and loving as was her norm. She had her two local grandkids over for sleepovers, and played Mah Jong with friends... As part of her follow up treatment, Wendy took oral Tamoxifen. As Tamoxifen was said to increase a woman's chance of having a gynecologic cancer, she was monitored regularly with exams and ultrasounds.

It was during one of these ultrasounds that her doctor saw "shadows" surrounding her ovaries. As Wendy had long suffered with ovarian cysts, and was past the age of menopause, her doctor suggested a hysterectomy with a dual purpose: to remove the source of her discomfort and to properly diagnose what he thought might be ovarian cancer.

The surgery was performed on October 21, 2001, when Wendy was 57 years old, just two years after her breast cancer diagnosis. Her OB/GYN and surgeon, who is a renowned gynecologic oncologist, came out after the surgery and informed us that she did, indeed, have epithelial ovarian cancer which had spread throughout her abdomen. They informed us that they had removed all visible signs of the cancer and that chemotherapy would be the next step in treatment. She was stage 3B.

Before she began chemo, Wendy was tested for the BRCA gene mutation and tested positive for BRCA1. This explained why she was diagnosed with not one, but both breast AND ovarian cancer. The fact that both cancers were diagnosed within two years was somewhat unusual. Immediately after Wendy's genetic results, her daughter, Heidi, tested negative, as did her sister, Cathie. Wendy's positive results were explained by her paternal grandmother and two aunts having suffered and died of breast cancer, all at a young age. It is believed that the BRCA mutation was passed to Wendy by her father.

Chemo began about three months after Wendy's surgery, and continued for about 9 months. The following year, she was considered to be "cancer free" (NED) and happily grew her hair back and proceeded with life.

Year two---- CA125 numbers had risen, so Wendy began again with chemo, but was being treated with a different course of drugs. Again, weird, horrible side effects, but no "symptoms" of the actual disease that she could discern.
Year three— the cancer had metastasized to her liver. Wendy was back on chemo. There were horrible side effects to this course of treatment, but she plodded along with the highest of hopes for a complete cure.

Year four--- another year, different chemo drug.

Year five--- the cancer had spread again, this time to her lungs. Wendy proceeded with yet another course of chemo. She was slowing down by this time, but had still not given up hope. With her fabulous hats and scarves, Wendy kept her teeth gritted and a smile on her face, and went into what would be her final course of treatment with renewed determination but a realistic view of what was happening.

It should be noted that Wendy was, as everyone is, very nervous and scared when she was first diagnosed with ovarian cancer and was told that she'd have to undergo chemotherapy treatment. After she went to an introductory "Chemo Class", she had "business cards" printed with her name and phone number. Wendy offered these cards to newly diagnosed ovarian cancer patients and acted as their "sole sister", offering information, guidance, and sometimes, simply a hug. You see, Wendy had collected miniature shoes since childhood, and had somewhat of a "fetish" about them… She helped many a frightened, sick woman through the terrible time when they were first diagnosed.

Towards the end of 2006, the cancer in her lungs and liver began to make itself known symptomatically. Wendy was sometimes short of breath and had intermittent pain in her chest. In December, as her liver began to shut down, Wendy became jaundiced and, while she did not verbalize the sad truth, knew that her life was ending. My dad and I did absolutely everything we could to keep her comfortable. She had a pump for pain, and sometimes when she was too weak to push the button for more medication, I would do it for her. My brother and aunt, as well as numerous friends, came to be with her to show their love and support.

Wendy Sheron died five years and two months after being diagnosed with ovarian cancer on January 16, 2007. She fought so hard and for so long. My last conversation with her included her asking me, "What will you tell the children?" I told her that I'd worry about that, and she just needed to do what she needed to do'. I told her that 'it was okay'.

Before her death, my Mom used to tell me that she wanted to be the Susan G. Komen of ovarian cancer, but she wanted to LIVE. Of course, that did not work out as hoped, but my husband and I became involved with the Georgia Ovarian Cancer Alliance, a nonprofit education and awareness organization, not long after she passed away. We both became Board members, and eventually, the organization (GOCA) hired my husband, Doug, to be its Executive Director. Six years later I'm very proud to say that Doug has grown the organization and made great strides in helping the women of Georgia to be better informed, better educated, and better prepared to deal with the horrible disease called ovarian cancer.

I'd like to think that Mom smiles down on us as she watches us live on as we try to honor her.

Chapter 4

What Are We Going to Do?

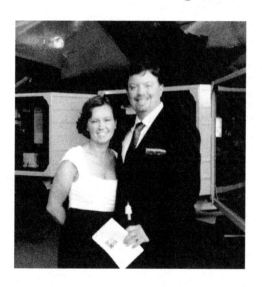

By Chris Baxter
(Husband of Virginia Baxter)

During the spring of 2012, my wife was suddenly diagnosed with Stage 3B Ovarian Cancer. As you can only imagine the thoughts that came into our minds ... What are we going to do? What does this mean? How did she get this? Why was this not detected in her last doctor's visit? The list goes on. She was rushed into surgery before we could blink. After, being diagnosed to three weeks later, having surgery for this life changing disease, we were in a complete whirlwind. Life as we knew it had come to complete standstill. However, we ended up at Northside Hospital, under the direct care of Dr. Gerald Feuer. He is a specialist in Ovarian Oncology and the World's Leading Robotic Surgeon.

Along the way we have had the opportunity to meet some really wonderful people. They have helped us so much from education on Ovarian Cancer to receiving treatment. One of those individuals is Doug Barron at the Georgia Ovarian Cancer Alliance. Upon the beginning of treatment at Northside each patient receives a "Bag of Hope". After my wife got hers I started digging in it and discovered a lot of great items in it that a cancer patient needs while undergoing treatment. Little did I know that this would lead into something far more than I could imagine. I had thoughts jumping into my head and felt the sudden urge to try to make a difference. I immediately called and left a message on Doug's voicemail and to my surprise he called me back, enthusiastically wanting to hear my plans.

I came up with a way to raise awareness and to help save a life that he never envisioned. I presented him with a boat wrap to travel across the country, mainly Georgia to help reach women and families that may never have the opportunity to know about early detection of this Silent Killer. We can reach outside the Atlanta area into the rural surrounding counties and bordering states for an outreach program that may never had come about without my wife becoming ill. Most victims of this disease come into the Atlanta area for treatment, the very same place that I will be traveling to.

Fast forward to four years later, here we are still traveling down the same road, however the cancer is holding off and we are waiting for the exciting five year anniversary. I am reaching farther into more communities than ever before. It has gone by so fast but just seems like yesterday when it all began. For those of you that have no clue there are any way to understand all the bumps in the road that we have traveled but the ones that have walked in our shoes can and will as they read on.

This has been an incredible journey and learning experience that as a caregiver I had no clue on beforehand. I am sure of one thing, everyone is different and we all handle these challenges with the upmost importance but when a loved one is suffering we just want to make it all go away. This cancer does not know how old you are, it just wants to attack you, do its damage and move on in hopes of not being caught. That is why it is the silent killer and where I come into the picture.

During the past four years I might not have saved a life single handedly, however, I have educated hundreds if not thousands of people with the most simple and easiest way out there, word of mouth. However the Georgia Ovarian Cancer Alliance has provided me with a great tool also, the Ovarian Cancer symptom card. I give these cards out all across the country and if you are like me and open up a desk drawer you will find hundreds of business cards inside. At some point you will need to clean that junk drawer out to make room for more clutter and when you do guess what? There is your symptom card, and what do you do with it? Trash it? Maybe, Read it again? Hopefully, or wait realize that you know someone, possibly a loved one or yourself that has the very symptoms listed on it then immediately take action. Voila, you have potentially saved another life from this deadly disease.

The scary thing is, me being a guy, I may know more than most women out there about ovarian cancer and definitely more than all the other men but the single most common thing I hear when I talk about it is" I go to my Dr. once a year for my checkup" Guess what? They don't check for ovarian cancer unless you are proactive or have a reason for them to do so. Educate yourself and your doctor. Early detection is the key.

Being a caregiver is probably harder to do that actually having the cancer and receiving the chemo treatment. You have to be the coach, the cheerleader, the counselor, the husband and even sometimes the doctor. Staying positive is so hard but you have be strong in order get your loved one stronger. This is very simple to say but we all know how difficult it becomes when you are weeks or even months into treatment. For most of us, treatment is six months to a year and a half if not longer with doctor visits that never end.

This is why my story has no closure and honestly it may never end because I am willing to be proactive for all the others out there and hope you will too. This is not cause that you follow; it is an extended family you become a part of because you meet so many people along the way during your journey.

Who would have thought that a fishermen would be part of this?

Chapter 5

The Journey

By Mary Bernier

This journey began in 1990 and we didn't realize how seriously it would impact the lives of my sister's daughter Mary Beth, myself and my daughter Emily. My sister Kate called late one evening and I will never forget the panic in her voice! They are calling it adenocarcinoma! What is that? What am I going to do! I can't die! I have two girls to raise. Kate was divorced but she was the glue that held our family together. She was artistic, caring and a beautiful person inside and out. The final diagnosis was stage 4 OVCA, a death sentence.

At that time the chemo was brutal, not to mention the cruel and violent vomiting that followed. Not any good anti-nausea drugs available-it was dehumanizing! Then she was subjected to a second look surgery, which was protocol at the time, it was a disaster! Her colon was perforated, and life would never be the same. Again, dehumanizing! The doctors just went about their business like it was just a regular day, but for our family it was life changing. She passed away a year after her diagnosis. She made me promise that a CA125 would be part of our yearly GYN exam. Her CA125 was off the charts when she was diagnosed-a definite marker for her, and at the time I had a normal CA125 in 1992 and 1993, and because the test was so expensive I was discouraged from having another. Of course, because there was no cancer on the maternal side of the family I was in the clear. Shame on me! When I had a yearly GYN visit in 1994, I knew something was wrong, but I was also unaware of the symptoms. I was tired, had a back ache, lost weight, and didn't have an appetite. As a busy working mother I thought this was normal. In June of 1994, I was diagnosed with Stage 3 OVCA, and my CA125 was off the charts! Never made my sons high school graduation.

Bummer! I not only had to tell my husband and children, but I had to tell my Mom and dad that they were probably going to lose another daughter to OVCA. This was surreal! How could this be happening! What a mess! I don't think my brain processed all the information, and I was so afraid! My Mom was with me when I had my first dose of chemo. I was so scared I can't even describe my feelings in words. Maybe later...

I had a wonderful surgeon and a wonderful oncologist. I was put into a clinical trial, which almost killed me, but I survived. During this time I met some wonderful women who were in the same situation as me. We formed a support group and that group became the Georgia Ovarian Cancer Alliance. We were all looking for answers. I remember one young woman in her early twenties came to our support group, and wanted answers and alternatives. She wanted to live and we couldn't help. I think that's when we went full speed ahead. The song at her funeral was "The Dance". Please take a Moment to listen to the words.

The Girls

Ginger was our fearless leader. We started our attack in her kitchen, no money, just crazy ladies wanting to make a difference. She was married to an attorney who helped establish our organization, bylaws and all that stuff. We depended on George, then he divorced Ginger and so divorced all of us. Susan's goal was to write a book and have it published. "No More Bad Hair Days" was published. Such a cute book full of humor and a celebration of life. Trudy was always there, a constant presence. As sick as she was she came to Washington to the OVCA National Conference. We ate lightly and took a taxi everywhere. Her cancer had metastasized. I can't imagine her pain. Then there was Judy who took out a 10,000 dollar life insurance policy on herself so her grandchildren would inherit more money. All she had to do was live two more years. AND SHE DID! So many wonderful women just to name a few.

We began working small booths at health fairs at local hospitals, a walk in Centennial Park, Cabaret Nights at the Alliance Theatre with a silent auction, a fashion show with Jeffrey Ellis. We also marched at the Capitol building in Atlanta for insurance companies to approve the CA125 test. The greatest evening was the night we sponsored Wit at the Alliance. Maggie Edson, The Pulitzer Prize winner for the play Wit, graced us with her presence. She told our story and captured the essence of who we were as ovarian cancer women. She truly made a difference in bringing awareness to our cause. We will be forever grateful!

In 2008, I had a recurrence of OVCA! 15 years later! Really! I had a colon resection and began chemo, AGAIN. This time the cancer had spread and I would be on a maintenance chemo forever. But that changed after my niece Mary Beth, my sister Kates daughter was diagnosed with OVCA in 2010. She was 30 years old. She travelled with an Olympic horse trainer and was in Europe. MB thought she had a colon problem but was sent home a very sick young woman. My Mom and my sister Beth were visiting us at the lake at the time, the visit was cut short and they flew back to Massachusetts. Mary Beth had late stage ovarian cancer. What a nightmare! What the hell! AGAIN!

Let me back up. We were all advised to have genetic testing. Of course, I had the gene and we are pretty sure Kate had the gene. MB's sister did not, my son did not, but my daughter did! Mary Beth did not have the test, but you know she had it. My daughter Emily was now high risk due to her BRCA deformity. Emily had a hysterectomy at age 29. Another nightmare! Would any woman want instant menopause at age 29? That's a story for another day! One thought that resonates with me is when she said to me one day, "Mom, Mary Beth saved my life." The BRCA gene was inherited from my father's side of the family. Thanks dad, but I still love you. Due to the gene, we have an 87% chance of breast cancer.

Mary Beth was married in 2014. We all went to New York and were featured on "Say Yes to the Dress". Her husband knew what he was getting into, but he loved her so much it didn't matter. She passed away in 2015 at age 35. I'm so conflicted because I feel we have done so much to raise awareness, and yet I'm so sad that it has afflicted my love ones before finding a cure. She will be buried at sea in Ogunquit, Maine in July. It's been a special place for our family forever.

Bob and I decided after my recurrence that we would buy a home on Lake Nottley in the North Georgia Mountains, where we would hope to retire one day. Sounds crazy, but it was fun. Now we needed a boat! Not only did my husband marry Kojak (I loved tootsie pops while I was bald and on chemo) but try boating with a wig! Great healing place. Lots of laughs! His support was so important to my well-being, I can't express in words how important and comforting it is.

That said, after 4 years on maintenance chemo I had had it! So I went to Dana Farber in Boston for a second opinion. That's where Mary Beth was being treated at the time. I was told that I would have to stop my chemo, let the disease progress so I could qualify for a clinical trial. WOW WHAT A GREAT CHOICE! However, I made the decision to stop the chemo. It was killing me anyway. *I am a faith filled person who truly believes in God's will for my life. I never asked for a cure. I have been cancer free for 3 years! WHO KNEW! THANK YOU LORD!*

Chapter 6

The Cruelness of Ovarian Cancer

By
Melissa D. Brock
Kayla Brock
Diana Brock
Karen (Sister)

Age Diagnosed: 46
Date Diagnosed: October 7, 2013
Epithelial Stage 3C serous Ovarian Cancer

My journey starts way before I was diagnosed with Ovarian Cancer. I had a tubal ligation back in February 1993. I went to my Primary Care Physician ("PCP") to have my yearly pap smear, on the fourth year of having an irregular pap smear my PCP referred me to a gynecologist specialist. The gynecological specialist does another pap smear, which comes back with irregular cells. I have irregular bleeding between periods so, in July 2012 the specialist does multiple tests, including transvaginal ultrasound. She said all test were negative and everything looked good.

A couple of months go by, and I start having a lot of gastrointestinal issues from heartburn to throwing up and even diarrhea and constipation. I also had dizziness with a lot of bloating and pain in the abdomen. I visited my local emergency room four times with these symptoms within a year. I always followed up with my PCP. In my medical records it showed that my maternal grandfather had breast cancer and prostate cancer. The doctors from the ER instructed me to lose weight, take some antacids and not eat within 2-3 hours before bed. In June 2013, I was feeling like I was pregnant. July 2013, it was time for my yearly pap smear, but my husband had a heart attack, so I put off going to the doctor.

In August 2013, I was hurting badly and was very sick. I followed up with my gynecologist. I told her I felt like I was pregnant and told her my symptoms, she looked in my file and saw that 15 months ago she had done a transvaginal ultrasound. She decided to do one that day. She saw a cyst on both of my ovaries. She ordered a CA125 blood test to check the amount of cancer antigen protein that was in my blood. A normal result would be a 35 or below. When I left the office that day I was very scared. I called my husband and talked to him and he made me feel better by

44

reassuring me that everything was going to be okay. A day went by and I did not hear from the doctor's office about my blood results. The next day I received a phone call at work on my cell phone. The doctor left a message for me to call her. I called her and she had set me up a CT scan for the following Tuesday, by Friday of that same week the doctor left another message for me to call her. I was at work so I went to my boss Laura and told her the doctor wants me to call her about my blood test results and the CT scan. I didn't want to be alone. Laura, my boss, told me to come into her office and close the door. I called Sharon, my doctor, she told me that CA125 came back at 356, which is very high. That the CT scan showed a 10 cm cyst on the left ovary and a 5 cm cyst on the right ovary.

She referred me to a gynecologist oncologist. She had four different doctors, I asked her who she would send her daughter to if she was in the same position I was in, and she said Dr. Jeffery Hines. He works out of Southern Regional in Riverdale. Sharon said he is a Christian man. I called Dr. Hines office to set up an appointment. My husband (Thomas), and my daughter (Diana) both went with me to see Dr. Hines. His nurse Susan took us to a room where there was a couch. Dr. Hines and Susan sat directly in front of us. He starts by telling me what was found on the CT scan. He never speculates that it might be cancer. He tells me I will need a hysterectomy, and possibly a debulking depending on what is found when he opens me up. He wants me to meet with a doctor to fix my umbilical hernia, and he gives me the doctor's name and number. Dr. Hines and Susan prayed with us that day before we left. I still did not know at this time that I had ovarian cancer.

I went by Southern Regional and pick up my CT scan disk, and the radiology report for the doctor who will be doing my hernia surgery. After receiving the CT scan and radiology report I headed to work. When I got there, I took a few minutes to read the radiology report. In the report the only thing that sticks out is the word metastasized to my liver and omentum. When I look up the word metastasized it means that cancer has spread to other areas of the body. I then take the report to my other boss Jessica, I wanted someone else to take a look at the radiology report. I wanted to make sure I was reading the radiology report correctly. I started to tear up because I was really scared now. Jessica told me "not to count my chickens before they hatch", I just giggled and wiped away my tears.

I made arrangements with my work to be out for 6 to 8 weeks for my hysterectomy. The big day was October 7, 2013, which is my husband and I's 24th wedding anniversary. I knew at that time I had cancer, but I had not told any of my family members. I just did not know what stage cancer it was at that time. In the morning of October 7, 2013, we got to the hospital, we checked in, they got me ready for surgery. Before surgery, Dr. Hines prayed with me. The doctor that was going to do my hernia surgery was sick, and unable to fix my hernia that day. I don't remember much, my family came in and kissed me. I do not remember anything that occurred, until I woke up in recovery nauseated and in pain.

I remembered biting my finger to dislocate the pain I was feeling. Once I was awake they took me to a room. My family came into my room in twos. Dr. Hines had come out and told them I had ovarian cancer while I was in recovery. I cried some, but it was not a shock to me. Dr. Hines came in later that afternoon to tell me what comes next. Dr. Hines said that the tumors disintegrated when he removed them. He had to remove the omentum and 2 liters of fluid, and I had a small node on my liver. He said I would do 18 rounds of chemotherapy after my incision healed. I don't think it felt real about the cancer at that time. My husband started pushing me to walk the halls at the hospital the day after surgery. I was so sore in my abdomen, I could barely walk. I had to get a port put in before I started chemotherapy. That was not a bad experience, it went well, and I was scheduled for chemo at

Southern Regional infusion center. That is where I met Daryl and Jackie, the nurses that took care of me for the next 18 weeks.

Daryl the chemo nurse was really nice. He explained everything to me as he accessed my port to draw blood to check my counts. He explained how the chemo might affect me from nausea to diarrhea, hair loss to my blood counts dropping. It doesn't hurt to get chemo, it's the after effects of chemo that hits you days later, and makes you feel bad. Psychologically, I thought I was prepared to lose my hair, but losing my hair was one of the hardest things I've ever experienced. I was losing another piece of myself. The first round of chemo was Carboplatin and Taxol for 18 weeks. I was hospitalized four times within those 18 weeks due to dehydration, and at one point I was septic. After this round of chemo, my CA 125 was an 8. Which was awesome!

During my first round of chemo Dr. Hines recommended I get genetic testing to see if I am BRAC1 or BRAC2. I had the test done and I am BRAC2. The genetic doctors traced it back to my maternal grandfather. Most likely he was BRAC2 and my mother must have been BRAC2 also. My two daughter will need to either be tested for this, or they will need to be proactive in making sure they follow up with their gynecologist regularly, so that they will never go through what I have been through. I have shared my results of this test with my cousins on that side of the family in hopes that they will be aware of their bodies. Most people do not know that men can carry this gene. My grandfather had both breast removed when I was a child because he had breast cancer.

Dr. Hines decided to do a CT scan and everything was clear. He then decided to do a maintenance chemo of Taxol and Avastin (Bevacizumab) for 12 months to make sure we got all the cancer. Avastin is a vascular endothelial growth factor inhibitor. My insurance company would not pay for the Avastin. They said if I have a reoccurrence that they would approve the use of Avasitn.

47

It's like they were playing with my life. I felt it was not fair, but I have learned that life is not always fair. During the treatment with Taxol, my CA 125 started to go back up and my hair started to grow back. I knew at that time that the chemo was not working, and the CT scan showed that I had several nodes on my mesentery of the small intestine.

I met with Dr. Hines and we decided on Avastin and Doxill (Doxorubicin) for 6 months. After 4 months of this round of chemo, the CT scan showed my cancer spread to both nodes of my liver, 2 tumors behind my spleen, 3 tumors in my pelvic area and some tumors in my left gutter. The chemo did not work at all, so my family and I decide I needed to go see another doctor for a second opinion. The other doctor said he would have followed the same path Dr. Hines was on.

So, my next round of chemo would be topotecan for four months. Had a CT scan, and it showed only three tumors in pelvic area, and some fluid and nodes in my right lung. Dr. Hines and I decided on Carboplatin and Gemzar for six rounds. Both chemo's one week, Gemzar the next and then off a week. After first round I ended up in the hospital with a white count of .6, red blood count of 7.5 and platelets a 7. I received two bags of platelets which I had an allergic reaction to, I got real hot and flushed and started to itch. After the itching I got really nauseated. The nurse gets me Benadryl and Zofran to make me feel more comfortable. I was supposed to get another bag of platelets but the doctors held off on it. I received two bags of blood, and my counts went up and I was able to go home.
On my next infusion of Carboplatin and Gemzar I had an allergic reaction to Carboplatin. My nurse just started the Carboplatin and I felt really hot, I started sweating, my chest got very tight and I could not breathe, my heart rate jumped to 150. The nurse stopped Carboplatin and started saline. She yelled for the head nurse to get the anaphylactic shock kit and administered

it to me. The head nurse hooked me up to the monitor, and after that she put oxygen on me at a 6 to see if she could get my oxygen level up. I was still having trouble breathing so they decided to call 911. The paramedics took me to the hospital which was next door. They basically did the same thing at the hospital that the nurses did at the infusion center. They were able to get my oxygen up to a 93 and they let me go home. During the allergic reaction I was so scared, I knew I was not getting enough oxygen and I felt like I was going to pass out.

This journey has been a challenge. I worked at my job until February 2016. My FMLA ran out so they had to let me go, it was sad and I was unsure of my future. I have always worked and built myself around my job. I really needed to concentrate on getting well, then I could go back to work. The fear I have every time I have a CT scan is sometimes so overwhelming. I have taken vacations once a year since I had been diagnosed. There were years in the past, that we as a family, had not gone on vacation. We take the time we have with our families for granted sometimes.

We as women need to listen to our bodies and if you feel something is wrong don't be embarrassed to get a second opinion, ask for a blood test and get a pelvic ultrasound. I've learned to listen to my body these past few years. Doctors always tell you not to google things on the internet, but if I would have, I may have been able to find what was wrong with me before it reach stage 3C. I cannot believe how my life has changed these past years.

I am enjoying my life now. I have my bad days, and cry buckets of tears. I met many people on my journey, and all of them have been a blessing. My favorite saying is "God's got this!" Life is short, so make the best of everyday; love, live, and laugh…..

Kayla Brock
(Daughter of Melissa Brock)
Why My Mother?

Imagine someone close to you just got diagnosed with cancer. How do you deal with it? Let's make it even more personal, it's your Mom. How cliché are these questions? There is no way that you could ever imagine your reaction to your Mom being diagnosed with cancer, at least not until it happens.

My Mom was diagnosed with ovarian cancer almost 3 years ago to this day. I can remember having so many questions about the "solution" for this "problem" that just arose in my life. See I am a problem solver, a thinker. In times of crisis I can compartmentalize my reactions to a particular situation. So when my Mom came to me to tell me she had ovarian cancer my first thought was not sadness, surprisingly, it was what do we do about this? I asked all the typical questions: "what stage?", "how long do you have to live?", "are you sure the doctor knows what they are talking about?", "what is the doctors plan to fix this?" Of course, my Mom didn't have any of these answers right off the bat, all she could tell me was she was going to see a cancer doctor that specialized in ovarian cancer.

My Mom will tell you how she was diagnosed and everything she has done to fight for this life she has. I am here to tell you about what my Mom's diagnoses means to me. You may think, what could your Mom having cancer do to you? When the strongest woman you know gets diagnosed with something like cancer, where she is given 5 years to live, you start to think about your life. My Mom is a fighter. Before cancer she was a fighter, but I just did not realize it as clearly before she was diagnosed with cancer. Watching her do whatever it takes to give herself just a little longer in this world has been a great inspiration to me. My Mom's diagnoses and battle with cancer has also brought me closer to God, and has strengthened my Christian walk. If cancer has done anything positive in my life it has shown me just what you can handle through faith and trust in the Lord.

Ultimately, when my Mom was diagnosed with cancer our family's life changed. Now there were doctors to go to on a regular basis and tons of medicine. Then how was the insurance thing going to work out, and what happens if Mom loses her job? A lot of things became unclear. The hold you thought you had on life starts to weaken. Personally the hardest thing was worry for me. I was away at college and could not be home with my Mom all the time. I worried about her health, both physically and mentally. I wanted to be there on those days where all she needed to do was cry on someone's shoulder. I now live in north Georgia with my husband and children, and still miss out on a lot of the treatments and physical struggles my Mom has. I want to leave you with a thought that I believe crosses everyone's mind when they are diagnosed, or have someone close to them diagnosed, with cancer... why me/them? I don't have an answer for you, but know that you are not alone.

Diana Brock
(Daughter of Melissa Brock)
The Caregiver's Side of Ovarian Cancer

My mother's name is Melissa Brock, my name is Diana Brock. I am going to tell you how it feels to be the care giver of a patient who has ovarian cancer. When I was 21 I got pregnant and from then on my mother was like my best friend. I am going to school to be in the medical field. She did so much for me when I was pregnant, and even to this day she does more for me than anyone else.

I knew my Mom was not feeling well, but my mother never really verbalized it. Within 15 months before she was diagnosed so much happened. My dad and I took her to the hospital four different times and they literally just told my mother she was to fat, and she needed to take better antacids. I never told her, but man did those ER doctors piss me off. I cannot tell you how many times it has taken me to just walk out the room, because I wanted to punch them. I knew something more was wrong with my Mom, I just did not know what the heck it was. Never in a million years did I ever think it would be cancer. In April, I got an amazing new job and I was getting ready to move out. My Mom begged me to not leave. She said she knew with whatever was upcoming for her health she would need me. And boy was she right. My dad had a massive heart attack at the end of July 2013. My Mom was in Florida visiting her half-sister when it happened. I called her and her sisters and she made her way back to Georgia.

September 9, 2013, is a day I will never forget. My mother never called my cell phone while I was at work, she always called my work number if she needed me. When she called my cell I knew something was wrong, and I just knew it would be bad. I answered my phone and walk to the back, during this time my employer knew my mother was having medical issues. She told me she was having to go see a gynecologist oncologist. When she said oncologist I swear my stomach dropped to the floor, and I felt sick and scared. I started to cry and my mother asked me to be her health care advocate. Meaning, I would take care of her because during this time where my dad was working he couldn't take days off, and was too far away to get to her quickly if she was taken to the hospital. I said yes and got off the phone and went and informed my boss what was going on.

On that day I left early because I had to drive to Griffin for class. I was getting ready to close when my boss told me to come to the back, she needed to talk to me. I was fired. No warning at all. They had no proof for the reason they fired me so they ended up paying part of my unemployment check. We did not know that this was actually a blessing in disguise, because now that I wasn't working I was going to be able to take care of my mother full-time.

October 7, 2013, was the day my mother was to have her hysterectomy. It was also the day we would find out if she indeed had cancer. The waiting for her doctor to come out and talk to us felt like years, but it was only hours. When he told us she definitely had cancer, it was one of the worse days of my life. I kept asking God, why in the world would you allow such an amazing selfless woman to have this? Why her? I needed her so much, and I was absolutely terrified I was going to lose my mother. We were told she was going to need chemotherapy, and that it would start after she got her port placed. She got out of the hospital two days before my daughter's first birthday.

I took my Mom to get her port put in, that was just the beginning of this new scary journey. She was to take Carboplatin and Taxol for her first chemo treatment. During this treatment she was hospitalized four times, one of those times was on Thanksgiving Day. This was really a scary time for us, her blood pressure went from 100/80, which is a good blood pressure, to less than 15 minutes later 80/50. She could barely hold her eyes open.

Now, if you understood my dad you would get why when things like this happened he felt the need to scream at her, and make everything worse. I was able to calm her down and get her doctor's number and he told us to get to the hospital. She ended up being almost septic. She was close to renal failure. My Mom tells me to this day, that I saved her life. My Mom having cancer was hard on everyone. Everyone had different ways of handling it. I know some people deal with things by being angry, but right now was not the time. I am not going to sugar coat anything. My dad was the biggest jerk ever and almost three years later he has just got so much worse. He tells my Mom she should just stop taking chemo. The doctor told my mother if she ever stops taking chemo she will be dead within 6 months. The chemo is what is keeping her alive!!! And I wanted her to stay alive.

53

Carboplatin and Taxol put my mother in remission for four months. The next couple of treatments did not work. Taxol for a year, Doxol and Avastin for 6 months, Topotecan for about 4 months, and now she is on Gemzar and Carboplatin. Through all the chemo treatments we've dealt with nausea and vomiting, diarrhea and constipation, hair loss to dehydration, to her counts being so low she needed blood and platelet transfusions. Since I am with her all day every day I am able to tell when something is really wrong. I know by what she eats in the morning if it is going to be a good day or a bad day.

I have learned to deal with her crying episodes, and her talking about her funeral. Her talking about her funeral is probably the hardest thing to listen to. Knowing that eventually we will be following her wishes. I can honestly say it's depressing and scary and it is my biggest fear to wake up and find her dead in her bed. I take videos and pictures of her and my daughter so when she is older and she asks about her, I can tell her about her Nana and I can show her.

My Mom has had people be cruel to her, my father being the worst, he is beyond selfish. He cares about his needs and his needs only. He doesn't care that my mother has 3 large tumors in her pelvic area and sex is uncomfortable for her, he just doesn't care. But he's not the only one. She can't walk through Walmart or Kroger like you and I can so she rides the little electronic chairs. I cannot tell you how many people make comments on how she is just riding it because she's fat.

When she lost her hair she wore head scarves, because it was cold and she wanted something on her head! We were at Ihop and some childish female said she shouldn't wear that because she's white. That is one time I did not just walk away, I told her head scarves are for everyone, and my mother doesn't have a choice, chemo has made her lose her hair and she does not want to wear a hat into a restaurant. When it comes to my Mom I am so over protective. My mother had an allergic reaction to Carboplatin on her second round of Carbo and Gemzar. I was not allowed to see her until 2 hours after the reaction had occurred because they were not sure if she was going to live. I was completed beside myself, I felt like I am her protector, she needs me with by her side.

While dealing with all this with my mother I have to be strong. But it is so hard. I have been battling severe depression since I was 13 and I am now 25. I also have severe anxiety, PTSD and borderline bipolar disorder. When my dad is a jerk to her, it's very hard for me to hold my tongue. I just want him to understand you cannot treat her the way you are treating her! From the outside looking in it does not look like he loves her. I know he does but it is questionable.

If I could give any husband/boyfriend advice when you find out the woman you are with has cancer, is to be supportive. Love her, be there for her, cry with her, laugh with her and enjoy her time. Same goes for anyone else honestly. We never know when that time will come to an end and you do not want to regret anything.

Karen
Why Not Me?
(Melissa Brock's Sister)

I am Melissa Brook's older sister, Karen. She asked me to write how I felt about her diagnosis of ovarian cancer. How it has affected me emotionally and physically.

I believe I should start where our story begins. I was one year old and 2 months when she was born. I called her my "Lissa Bug", because I couldn't quite say Melissa. She was my baby, but as we grew she became my best friend. Some thought we were twins because we were always together. As we grew we had our share of fights but we loved each other very much. Then, our little sister was born and Melissa became jealous and my attention moved to having another baby. That jealousy sometimes caused problems, but we survived it through loving each other unconditionally.

I have had Melissa as my very best friend for a long time, 50 years almost. So when she told me that she might have cancer, it ripped my heart out. The day she went into surgery was one of the longest days of my life. The whole time I sat in the waiting room praying that they were wrong, and if they were right dreading the days ahead not knowing how long I would have with her. Well, as you can see that they were right and I started wishing it was me. It sent me into a depression that I thought would end my life.

So, she started chemo and I started praying for her cure. After the first round of chemo we thought that she went into remission, but when the chemo stopped the cancer did not. This news ripped at every fiber of my being. I didn't know what I would do if this cancer took my sister. Death had already taken our mother, and that I thought would kill me, but this was worse.

Melissa would then have a test done to see if the cancer was one that passed through our family. It turns out that she is Brach 2 positive, which was passed down through our mother's side of the family. So I had the test done too. I had the same results, so now I had to take precautions so I could live to take care of her, her daughters and her grandchildren. I had a hysterectomy in 2014, and now have mammograms every six months. It tears at my soul every day that she suffers, but I am thankful that she is still here, and I get to talk to her every day. I am not looking forward to the day the Lord takes her home, but I praise Him for every day she is with me. My sisters are my heart and the thought of one of them not being here scares me to death.

So, this is just a little piece of how I feel about this situation. Since, my mother died I am the one that takes care of the family. I am the one that everyone turns to, so maybe that is why it's not me that has the cancer. Maybe God has a plan for me, but I still wish it was me.

Chapter 7

Our Story

By Robert Carey
(Husband of Patricia Carey)

The beginning of my story is either seven years ago, 2009, 2008, 2003, or earlier, maybe even 1955, that is the year I met Patricia. You see my story is our story, Patricia and I. Patricia and I met in high school, she was 14 and I was 15. We were together until her departure from this plane in 2009.

The life and the cancer journey we took was together, we did everything together so when I tell my story it is really the story of the two of us and our family. I am not sure when the ovarian cancer story started but it was labeled and the journey began in 2003 in the doctor's office. We knew before then that there was something seriously going on within her body, but we did not know what it was nor did any of the many doctors that treated Patricia.

I remember the doctor just before we were told that the diagnosis was cancer, ovarian cancer, was the only doctor I heard say, "I am not sure of what I am seeing so I want you to see a Gynecologic Oncology. She recommended someone and made the telephone call to the doctor's office to get Patricia in as soon as possible. Neither one of us slept very much for the next two nights as we waited for the appointment time. There were all sorts of thoughts running around in our heads. Some even coming out of our mouths to be shared.

Prior to the appointment the doctor reviewed Patricia's file and ordered additional tests. The day of the appointment he did his exam (I was in the exam room sitting behind a curtain). When the doctor completed the exam, we then moved to his office.

We were among the last of his patients for the day, so I knew the news we were about to hear was not going to be what we wanted to hear. I held Patricia's hand. The doctor told Patricia what we did not want to hear…cancer, ovarian cancer. At that Moment our lives changed and the ovarian cancer journey began. Six years of doctor visits, examinations, testing, blood draws, X-rays, Cat Scans (and other scans of her body), operations, chemotherapy and radiation, emergency room visits, various doctors, specialists, including Naturopathic Practitioners for consultation and opinions.

As the journey progressed I was to discover how little most people knew about ovarian cancer. The many things I had never heard of or thought about doing, that I learnt to do. I remember several times explaining the little I knew about the disease, and then hearing some of the recommended treatments, medicines, and herbs that were offered to Patricia. There was little or no research to support what was being suggested and recommended.

I found myself becoming jaded, frustrated, and angry, depressed that there was no one or any medicine that would halt the progression of the disease and cure it, to cure my love, and make her cancer free. There were Spiritual leaders and Practitioners we sat with for meditation and prayer. We had practiced meditation for several years but now we became stronger in our collective and individual meditation practice. I know it played a huge role in our journey and continues to support me today.

I remember at one of Patricia's CAT scan appointments sitting with her, because she suffered from mild claustrophobia so my presence helped her through the procedure. The cameras slowly rotated around her taking X-ray images and converting them to pictures, which along with the technicians I was able to view on the monitors. Of course, I did not know what I was seeing, except there were pictures of the inside of my love. The doctor thought this would give him more information about what was going on, and how to manage Patricia's treatment and medications making adjustments as needed. I knew she was scared, so was I, but I felt I had to put on a brave face for her and for me.

If I let her see me cry, and I did feel like I would. That would not be helping her. I knew she knew I was scared and concerned, we talked about it in many ways, many times. There were people Patricia talked with and I was happy about that, but there were not people I talked with, that I felt I could go into detail about what was happening inside of me. Many times I could not find the words to express my feelings out loud, to talk about what Patricia was going through, what we were going through and what I was going through.

You probably have noticed that I am saying we as I tell this story. That is because most visits to the doctor's office included me. I am not sure when this started but whenever possible I accompanied Patricia to the doctor's office and sat with her in the examination room. I believe it started in Florida in the eighties, and continued from there to New Jersey and then to Georgia. I believe there were early signs all along the way.

There are many parts to this story and I will share with you in the coming stories about stops/lessons/experiences along on the journey, on the road, observations in the waiting rooms, visits to emergency rooms, conversations with nurses, the doctors, medical technicians, staffers, conversations with people in the chemo-labs, the hundreds of needles to draw blood and give medications, and the support groups.

There are the other stories to be told of personal changes–my life-roles as a care-giver, reducing billable working hours, sleeping, eating, and drinking habits. And perhaps, the hardest, learning to be one to the love of your life with no experience.

Chapter 8

The Unimaginable—
My Little Girl has Ovarian Cancer

By Nicole Carter
(Mother of Mary Tipton Carter)

"Please pick up, please pick up, please pick up." I was driving home from the office. It was the day we had to tell our 8 year old daughter that she had been diagnosed with ovarian cancer. Finally, our neighbor answered the phone. I was crying hysterically. "Can I please come to your house and get myself together? I can't go home like this. And do you have whisky?" Our neighbor, Danielle, is also the mother of Mary Tipton's first and best friend, Mary. I parked in our driveway and fled down the street to Danielle's house before anyone in our house might see my car. She opened the door and I collapsed in her arms. "My baby. My baby, how can this be happening to my baby? How am I supposed to tell her she has cancer?"

It was one week to the day that we had found out ourselves. Mary Tipton had been to our beloved pediatrician, Dr. Thomas, for an ear infection. Two days later, I crept into the room she shared with her sister to wake her up for school. Certainly the antibiotics had kicked in by now and she would be ok for class. But, when I put my hand on her forehead she was on fire. My children tease me – rightfully so – that I take their temperature too often. But this time, I knew it wasn't just a case of me having cold hands. MT's temperature was almost 103 - too high for two days of antibiotics in her system. She woke up and said her stomach hurt. She vomited the ibuprofen we gave her for fever. So we called Dr. Thomas and made an appointment for that afternoon.

By the time we got to the doctor's office MT was the sickest I had ever seen her. White as a ghost and hunched over in pain, grasping her left side, she could barely walk. Dr. Thomas decided quickly that MT needed to get to the hospital. He called the children's hospital and told them we were on our way. I called my husband and asked him to come meet us. The assumption was either appendicitis or a nasty virus.

We were rushed to a room and the nurses immediately drew blood. Then we were whisked away to an ultrasound exam room. The movie "Mulan" was playing in the ultrasound room. To this day, that movie makes me feel like I'm going to vomit. The ultrasound technician told us she found an "abnormality" on Mary Tipton's ovary. Wait, what? She is 8 years old. How can that be? Then she told us MT would need another ultrasound in a little while. And with that, we were taken back to our ER room.

The ER physician told us that MT's blood tests indicated she had mononucleosis. Again, what? She is 8 years old. There is no smooching of the boys at 8 years old. Apparently, water fountains are the most common source of mononucleosis. We all get exposed to it, but as long as our bodies are otherwise healthy, we fight off the mono virus and never know the difference. But, our little girl was fighting cancer so the mononucleosis had taken its toll. Her spleen was enlarged. And thank God it was. Her spleen was large enough to crowd her growing ovarian tumor. Every oncologist we have seen has told us that the mono led to early detection of her cancer. Who ever thought we would be thankful for mono? But we are.

Then the ER doctor told us they suspected Mary Tipton's ovary was twisted and "torsing" – meaning it was twisting back and forth – and causing abdominal pain. Since the ovaries are part of the reproductive system, this is considered an emergency and MT would need surgery post haste. The doctor told us the surgery would be fairly minor – a laparoscopic procedure that should only take about 30 minutes. They would untwist her ovary and she would have a follow up ultrasound in 6 weeks. It should all be fine.

Three very long hours after MT was taken to the operating room the surgeon came to see us. She was holding photographs. Dr. Glasson told us she found a "mass" on Mary Tipton's left ovary. She told us she had removed Mary Tipton's ovary along with the mass. Our baby was now missing an ovary and we had no part in that decision. That is when I started to really feel helpless. With all the calm I could muster, I asked the question that no parent ever wants to ask about their child. "Is it cancer?" Dr. Glasson told us she was not sure, we would have to wait for pathology.

Dr. Glasson came to Mary Tipton's hospital room on a Friday morning. I had barely slept on the little sofa at MT's bedside – I'd spent the night praying, silently crying, begging God to not let MT have cancer. My husband and I followed Dr. Glasson into the hallway. She led us to some chairs in the nurse's station and asked us to sit down. Honestly, I don't remember exactly what she said. But she told us pathology indicated the mass was malignant. They had identified ovarian dysgerminoma, but would need to run further tests to determine if there was more than one type of malignancy in the mass. I asked her to write it down. Dr. Glasson pulled out her business card and wrote "ovarian dysgerminoma" on it. I still carry that card in my handbag. No idea why, but I can't seem to take it out of that little side pocket. Perhaps it's a reminder of what we went through and when I look at it occasionally it makes me thankful for where we are now.

We had to wait a month to start chemotherapy so that MT could recover from surgery and mono. The night before we checked into the hospital for port implant surgery and her first round of chemo, MT and I were getting settled into bed when she turned her sweet face to me and said, "Mama, I feel like I am too little for this to happen to me." It shattered my already broken heart.

There is no way to prepare for the onslaught of chemotherapy. Mary Tipton was brave, actually far braver than we expected she could be. But, dear Lord, she was sick.

It is important to remember that this is only one chapter. One chapter of this book – there are so many, too many, other stories of pediatric ovarian cancer. One chapter in our Mary Tipton's life – she has many more chapters to live, and for that we give thanks to God.

Chapter 9

Through Ovarian Cancer
I Built a Solid Foundation with God

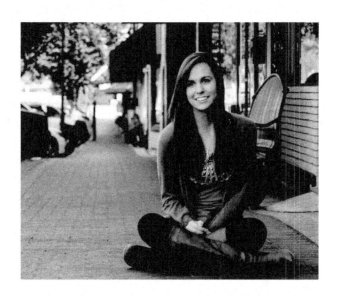

By Emily Coughlin

A lot of people think cancer is about the things that are lost; our ovaries, our hair, our health. But I like to focus on the things that I found. Through cancer, I found God, a better understanding of life, and in many ways, I found myself. My story started when I was in the eighth grade. I was a pretty average pre-teen; I got good grades, crushed on boys, was incredibly awkward (weren't we all). I would like to focus on was how healthy I was. I'm sure most people know by now that anyone can get cancer; you can be in perfect health but that doesn't just magically make your cells immune to uncontrollable division. I want my story to reiterate this fact, because I'd say I was in the best shape of my life at the time of my diagnosis. But I want to start a couple months prior to that.

Around the time of spring break in the eighth grade I started having sharp pains in my lower sides. At first they were very spread out so I just ignored it. They started to become more frequent and the pain became sharper, but they would also move around. Sometimes my right side would hurt, sometimes my left, sometimes even my back. I finally told my mom about them and she was confused by the movement and said we should wait to see a doctor because they might go away. They quickly got worse and were keeping me awake at night. I vividly remember the worst time, I got no sleep and was in the most pain I had ever experienced before, and it lasted for several hours. I went downstairs to take some Tylenol but had trouble getting back up the stairs, so I stayed on the couch for a while. Eventually I decided to give it another try, made it halfway up to a turning point in the stairs and had to stop there, doubled over in pain. I laid on the stairs for a while before making my second attempt, which got me all the way back to my bed. I thought about waking up my mom, but decided that it would be pointless to bother her about pain she could do nothing about, an idea I was going to have to get used to.

The summer after eighth grade was pretty busy. Every day I had cross country practice early in the morning and basketball practice right after that. Despite all that physical activity, I still seemed to be gaining weight right in the lower pooch of my stomach. I thought this was weird but brushed it off as not eating healthy enough. One day I was laying on my living room floor playing with my dog, Ziggy, when my mom first noticed my pooch. She too thought it was weird that I'd be gaining weight, especially in such a concentrated area. She asked to feel it and knew right away that something wasn't right. It felt hard as a rock. She immediately picked up the phone and made a doctor's appointment.

The day of my appointment started out as a regular summer day for me. I went to both of my practices, rode home with my friend Mandy like I did every day, and went swimming with two more friends. My mom arrived at the pool to take me to the doctor, I said goodbye and that was it. Looking back, I find it funny that I had no idea what was about to happen. I'm just hanging out with some friends, about to go discover the cancerous tumor that would change my life forever. I don't even think I told anyone what I was going to the doctor for. At that point I didn't think anything was serious, I hadn't even considered the possibility of a tumor.

We arrived at the office and it was a place I'd never been to before, filled with people I'd never met. But very soon all of these people would know who I am. My doctor walked in, introduced herself, asked about the problem, and asked me to lie down so she could feel it. As soon as her hand touched my stomach, I could feel a jolt of surprise run through her arm as she let out a slight, concerned "Oh." She left and returned with a man and an ultrasound machine. We just happened to schedule my appointment on a Thursday, the one day that the ultrasound man was in the office. I'd say that ultrasound lasted for about five minutes before they decided to send me to get an "emergency CT scan." They told me it was probably just a cyst and this was just a precaution. I'm not sure if she knew better and was just trying to make me feel reassured, or if she truly was hoping for the best. Either way, it worked; I was totally chill, just going with the flow. I'm sure my mom was very much the opposite, already running through the worst possibilities. We made our way over to the hospital, got my CT scan and entered into the first of many periods of waiting for results.

The doctor who found the mass recommended that I go see a certain oncologist. That oncologist was on vacation for another two weeks, but she said he was definitely worth the wait. And man, am I glad I waited. I'll talk more about him later, but this oncologist not only saved my life, but he actually made cancer somewhat enjoyable, and he has turned out to be one of my life's greatest mentors and role models. Anyways, he was nice enough to come back from vacation a little early to meet me and get started with this surgery process. He told me he thought it was something called a teratoma, which is actually one of the creepiest things in the world. Teratomas are tumors made up of different tissues and sometimes they include weird stuff like teeth, bones, hair and sometimes even eyes. Super creepy. On the bright side, teratomas are usually benign, so that was a good sign. But there was still a chance that it might be something cancerous.

I tried not to think about the possibility of cancer too much, but sometimes I couldn't help it. I'd think about it at night a lot instead of sleeping, one night in particular. It was really late; I had been up thinking for a couple hours. Usually, I forced myself to stay optimistic, but that night I was running through all the worst possibilities in my head. I think that was the first night that it really hit me that I might have cancer, and that this might only be the beginning. Maybe I was just scared and assuming the worst, but I really had a strong feeling that this thing inside me was cancer. Spoiler alert, it was. I was feeling helpless and overwhelmed, and I decided to turn to God. This decision was definitely something new for me. I didn't grow up in church, I had been attending a youth group for a couple years, but I was only going for the social aspect and never paid much attention to what was being said. But that night it felt like my best and only option. I started talking to God about how scared I was, which the first time I admitted that to myself was also. I realized this wasn't something I was going to be able to do on my own.

I told God that I needed Him to help me through it, and that I trusted whatever He was doing. I don't know how to explain it, but somehow everything made sense in that moment. God gave me so much understanding and wisdom beyond myself, and I knew that I had to commit my life to God. I started to feel extremely overwhelmed, but no longer with fear, now it was with the Holy Spirit. I felt an indescribable presence in my room and just started sobbing. I sat on my knees in my bed with my face down in the comforter, tears flowing. I told God that no matter what came of this, I would always follow Him. I understood that His plans were far better than my own, and I understood that all I needed to do was surrender my control, and He would make everything alright. I told God, "I want what you want." If you want me to be cured by the surgery, I want that too. If you want me to have cancer and go through chemotherapy, I want that too. If you want to take my life, I want that too. I give my whole life, whatever is left, to you. I could feel the presence in my room concentrated at the end of my bed, like God was just sitting there, so calm. There I was face down on my bed, crying and completely broken. And there was God, just sitting with me. It was then that I felt what can only be described as an intense relief. It was like God was literally taking all of my worries away, physically taking them off of my shoulders and into his arms. Ever since that night I knew that everything was going to be just fine, and that I'd never be alone. What could I possibly have to fear if God is in control?

On the morning of my surgery I was cool as a cucumber, unlike my mother who was as worried as any mother would be. I really was just thinking I wanted to get this surgery over with so I could eat food again (I had to fast for 12 hours before). A couple of years after all this cancer stuff blew over a little; I actually became an intern for Dr. Green and got to observe a lot of his surgeries. I would give anything to have been in the room observing my surgery because I can only imagine the looks on everyone's faces when it became clear that I didn't have a teratoma, but in fact had a cancerous yolk sac tumor. Dr. Green would tell my parents a few hours later that he could tell it was cancer just by looking at it. Another cool thing about my surgery was that I originally started out on the fancy new robot thing, but my abs were too hard for the robot to cut through, so the rest of my surgery had to be done unexpectedly by hand. Just a quick brag for my abs of steel, may they rest in peace because they haven't made an appearance since 2011.

After I woke up from surgery, some friends came to visit me. I found out later that my friends were told that I had cancer before I even woke up, I was kind of confused why they were acting weird and sad (but also just confused in general because of the morphine). I was told the news the next morning, right before I left the hospital. I was all packed up and ready to go when Dr. Green came in and dropped the bomb. But I really didn't feel very bombed, maybe because I was still pretty doped up. While he was explaining more, I noticed that the nurse standing behind him in the corner was crying, which really caught me off guard. I remember wondering whether I should be crying, although I didn't feel the urge to. While writing this part of my story, I asked my mom about that morning. She said everyone in the room was holding back tears and waiting to see how I would react. They were all utterly surprised when all I had to say was "Okay, so what do we do next?" I really think that at this point, I was not in control of anything. Everything was God. He was working through me, my reactions, my emotions; he had it all under control. I am not some incredibly strong and stable person on my own. I'm sure that if I hadn't surrendered my life to God, I would have been a worried mess. But my mind was so clear, and so calm that I was ready for anything because I knew God knew exactly what he was doing, so I just let him do his thing.

Dr. Green was confident that my tumor was cancerous, but that was about all the information he could give for a while. I had to wait a couple of weeks for lab results to process to find out how serious it was and what kind of treatment I would need. I joked about the wait to my mom saying the suspense was "killing me," but she didn't think it was as funny as I did. I wasn't afraid of what Dr. Green was going to say, it was like God put this worry-free shield on my brain and I was just ready to go in there and talk game plan. On results day, he told us that it was definitely cancer, and it hadn't spread outside my ovary but I was still going to need pretty aggressive chemotherapy. I asked him if I was going to lose my hair, and he said yes, probably. I looked over at my mom thinking "Man, we better do some hat shopping," but she was tearing up so I thought maybe that wasn't the time for a shopping pitch. I asked him if I was still going to be able to play sports, assuming he would say yes but it would be difficult. I was ready to put up with struggling harder than everyone else. But I was taken by surprise when he said no. That's when I cried. Losing my hair was fine, but no basketball? That's just cruel. So I was going to need three rounds of a regimen called BEP, which is a combination of three drugs called bleomycin, cisplatin, and etoposide. I would go to chemotherapy for about 4-6 hours every day for a week, and then have two weeks of treatment only on Monday, then the cycle would repeat. Since I would be getting drugs administered every day, I needed to get a pickline, which was this set of tubes that stuck out of my arm for three months where the machines attached. Those things were unbelievably annoying. Not only was it just the fact that I had tubes flapping out of my arm all the time, but they couldn't get wet. That meant awkward showers and no swimming, which especially sucked because I started chemo in July.

In the beginning of treatment, I continued to go to cross country practice thinking I could just do some light jogging and it wouldn't be a problem. Well I have never been more wrong. I remember the morning after day three of chemo I only made it through the first ¼ mile of the warm-up before feeling like I was definitely going to die, so that was an eye-opener. It was near the end of week two that the side-effects really started to kick in. Side-effects are what make chemo so terrible. You are essentially spending hours a day flowing poison throughout your body, so side-effects pop up all over the place. The worst for me were nausea and fatigue. Everything I ate made me want to throw up. Eventually all food started to taste like chemo, which is hard to describe. And I never wanted to eat anything. One day my mom actually yelled at me for not eating because it was starting to get dangerous and she was getting worried. Side note, my mom was a superhero through it all and I couldn't have done it without her. Anyways, I also was so tired all the time. Walking 100 meters was pretty much my limit before having to sit down and rest because I felt so heavy and dizzy. I felt like I was always hunched over from the combination of nausea, pain and tiredness. I also had some smaller side-effects including sores in my mouth and on my hands and feet and labored breathing. By the end of chemo, I actually lost most of my sense of taste all together. A lot of chemo patients experience changes or temporary loss of taste, but mine was different. There's this thing that runs in my family that causes some of us to not be able to smell, and obviously that affects taste a little too since they're so connected. Well I already couldn't smell, and had a hindered sense of taste before treatment, but chemo caused me to lose most of what was left of my taste. Unlike other people, mine wasn't coming back. But on the bright side, food didn't taste like chemo anymore near the end. Five years later I still haven't regained my taste.

One day in particular was the low point of my chemo treatment. I was feeling indescribably sick. I felt so weighed down that I didn't want to move at all. My arms and legs felt a hundred pounds each. So I just laid there in my bed, feeling like my stomach had either just torn in half or was about to make its way up my throat and outside my body. For a few minutes I thought it just wasn't worth it. I really just wanted to die, no person should experience this. It wasn't worth it. I still had weeks left of chemo, there's no way I could make it through feeling like this. I just wanted to give up. But suddenly I started visualizing my life years ahead, many years, and how much impact I could have. I could help other people going through cancer. There are so many people that would take on cancer alone, without God, when they don't have to. I needed to tell people to turn to God. Those people need me to guide them. Whoa, those thoughts were not my own. I was slipping, and God pulled me right back up and showed me that those moments of suffering were not the end of the line for me. He showed me that he has so much more for me to do. I needed to stay strong and make it through this, because there would be people in my future that need me. And so with strength and understanding from God, I persevered.

All this talk of symptoms has gotten me a bit ahead of myself. Backing up a little, to the Tuesday of week two of treatment, I spent the night at my best friend Blakeley's house. I planned on waking up at 5 a.m. to go to practice just to be there, maybe help out here and there. When I woke up, a significant amount of my hair had fallen out while I was asleep and got tangled into the mother of all messy buns. It was so bad I couldn't even get the hair tie out of my hair, and I started to get really frustrated and upset that the hair wasn't cooperating and I was going to be late to practice. I called my mom to come pick me up and instead of practice we went home to try to sort out the mess, but it turned out to be way worse than I thought. I sat on the couch and my mom sat behind me trying to save whatever hair she could, but it all just kept falling out the more she tried to undo the knot. I got so frustrated that my hair wouldn't stay attached to my head while coming to the realization that I was going to be bald very soon, and for the second time in this cancer journey, I cried. I cried a lot. A part of it was because I didn't want to lose my long hair, but I really think most of it was just anger at that stupid knot. My mom told me recently that that morning was one of the hardest for her. She said that she was sitting behind me, also frustrated with the stupid knot, but also crying, and trying to cry as quietly as possible. I think it was hard for her seeing all of it finally get to me. She ended up having to cut out the mega knot leaving me with short, chopped up, patchy hair. I want to take a moment here to appreciate my mom. She was such an incredible supporter and caregiver, I couldn't have done it without her. I can't imagine being in her position and watching your child suffer, but having to maintain a positive facade, but she did and she did it so well.

Normally, I would ride home with my friend Mandy and hang out at her house after cross country practice. Once the knot was cut out, and I settled down, I was ready to go on with my day, so I went over to Mandy's house. I let her go crazy on my hair with a pair of scissors since it was already a hot mess anyways, at least we could have some fun with it. That night at church turned out to be a head-shaving party. My youth pastor, Billy, did the honor of shaving my head and gave me a great Mohawk first, of course. After he finished, he decided he was going to shave his head too and even let me do it. After Billy, some of my friends decided to shave their heads too, and eventually all the boys there (and me) were bald, and all the girls had shaved a patch off the bottom of their heads. I feel incredibly lucky for such a great group of people to share that moment with. I think without those people, shaving my head could have been pretty depressing. But the head-shaving party was anything but depressing, everyone there had a blast and I didn't even care that I lost all my hair because I was having so much fun.

The first day of high school is generally a pretty nerve-wracking experience. I was already nervous, but then there was also that slight added factor of also being bald. My advice to anyone worried about the hair loss aspect of cancer is to just have a sense of humor about it. I think one of the worst times to have to lose all your hair as a girl is in school. But whether it's elementary, middle, or high school, people are just searching for reasons to make fun of others in order to make themselves feel better. High school especially is one of the most judgmental places on earth. But I eventually embraced being bald and made it something I was proud of, even though some people weren't able to accept it just yet. My boyfriend at the time broke up with me not long after my hair fell out. He did it at the end of lunch one day, right before I left school to go to chemo. A lot of people hear my story and think it's so sad that I had to start off high school bald but honestly, it was pretty fun. I used to ask girls to borrow their hairbrush, just to mess with them. And most people paint their bodies for football games, but I let people paint my head. I was really looking forward to being Charlie Brown for Halloween, but unfortunately I had grown out a buzz cut by then so I had to settle for G.I. Jane.

The first week of school, however, I had not yet embraced my baldness and was wearing a wig to school. Only a few people knew I was bald or had cancer at all, most people thought I just went blonde over the summer. On the second day of school I was getting really fed up with how itchy my wig was, so I lifted it up in the front, scratched my head, and put it back down without even thinking. I looked up and saw a boy across the room that saw it all. His eyes were wide and his jaw was on the floor, he didn't know what the heck he just saw. But after that I said screw it, wigs are itchy; I'm sticking to my beanie. That was when I basically, indirectly, outed my cancer.

My favorite bald story of all is twin day. Most high schools have different theme days during homecoming week, and one of ours was twin day. I was joking with a friend before an assembly that the only person in the school who could really be my twin was our bald principal. I wasn't actually serious but he said I should ask him, the worst he could say is no. Ironically, he was the first person we saw while walking into the gym. So I asked him, assuming he would laugh it off and say no. Not only did he agree, he even brought me a matching tie and pair of sunglasses. Everyone thought it was great, we got first place and a ton of candy, but more importantly, that was the first day I went bald all day at school and it was pretty liberating. After that I didn't care so much about wearing hats or what people thought when I didn't.

That month I was also voted to be on homecoming court, which was a really nice thing for my class to do. I decided to go out on the field bald instead of wearing a wig, and I honestly have never felt more beautiful in my life. And the great thing about that night was the chance to raise more awareness for ovarian and childhood cancer. I got interviewed by a radio station and a T.V. news station, reaching a lot of people who had never heard of someone so young getting diagnosed with ovarian cancer.

The process of finishing up chemotherapy really showed me how many people cared about me. My chemo nurse, Elizabeth, who was amazing and super helpful throughout my treatment, brought me balloons and cupcakes on my last day of chemo. My friends threw me a surprise party, which I didn't even know was for me until five minutes into it because it was on my friend's birthday so I thought it was for her. There were about fifty people at that party to celebrate my cancer victory, which was incredibly heart-warming. Having cancer in high school is weird, because your peers don't exactly know how to act towards you. A lot of people backed away, maybe because they thought I needed space or time to deal with such a big thing, but that wasn't the case. I had a few friends stay close through it all, they even came to chemo to keep me company sometimes. But for the most part, other people didn't know how to treat me or talk to me so they just didn't. So seeing all those people show up to support me showed me that people did actually care, they just didn't know how to show it.

Things were slowly getting more and more back to normal. My symptoms were dying down, I was going to school more, and I even started going to basketball practice again. But let's be real, my life is never going to be normal. One day at school I was standing in the lunch line and looked down to see that my arm was purple. I thought that was strange, but food is more important (especially since I could finally eat again without feeling sick) so let's finish lunch and then worry about my discolored limbs. I sat down at my usual table with my friends and started to eat. Everyone got silent and it went something like this:

Kiersten said "Emily..."

"Yeah?"

"Why is your arm purple?"

"I don't know." Bites into food.

"Go to the nurse."

"But I'm hungry."

"I'm taking you to the nurse right now."

And that's the story of how I ended up in the emergency room with a blood clot in my subclavian artery. I stayed at the hospital overnight on a heparin drip (a blood thinner) and was given a prescription for six months of Coumadin (another blood thinner) and would need to have my blood drawn once a week for those six months (fun, right?). Well that's all fine, all things I can deal with. But I soon found out that you can't play physical sports (aka basketball) while on blood thinners due to the risk of head injury and brain hemorrhage. I thought that once I finished my treatment that it would be over and done with. I beat cancer, I won, let's move on with life and be normal again. I had no idea what was ahead of me. This setback was just a glimpse into what would be a five-year long fight to be healthy again.

The next few months consisted of several trips to the emergency room for various reasons. For example, when February rolled around I thought I was ready to start running again, but I soon figured out that Bleomycin likes to tear up your lungs and leave you with asthma. I thought I was just super out of shape, but some constricted bronchioles and another trip to the ER proved it was a little more serious than that. And just like that, there goes track season.

Just as one problem started to get under control, a new one would pop up. Next was back pain, which turned out to be something called a Pars defect in my L4 vertebrae, I needed a few months of physical therapy for that. Not only was I not able to participate in any summer practices, I was barely able to do much of anything. The pain made it pretty uncomfortable to walk a lot or go from sitting to standing. And as if that wasn't enough, a month or two later was about the time that the worst side-effect of all started. This is one that would later take me out of school, and one that I still struggle with five years later. Chest pain. Idiopathic, undiagnosed, frustrating as hell chest pain. At first it was just sometimes, coming in little pain bursts. Imagine just sitting in class and all of a sudden getting a deep, sharp pain in your chest and all you want to do is lay down.

Usually, I would just rush out the door and go lay down in the hallway, which caused a lot of awkward confusion both from my teachers and hallway pedestrians. But after a while I learned to just stay put and tough it out until the pain died down because I didn't want to draw attention to myself. If it got bad enough or long enough I would go to the nurse and lie down and often even go home. But the skill of toughing it out still comes in handy because I still get those bursts of chest pain all the time. The pain gradually got worse and eventually I was in a constant state of dull, uncomfortable chest pain and would still get sharp pains at random on top of it. I went to multiple doctors, about 3 different types, and had a ton of scans trying to find out what was going on but none of them could find a definitive reason. One doctor thought it might be my gallbladder, so I got some test done to test the function of my gallbladder and it showed that it wasn't functioning properly, so I had surgery and it was removed. It turned out that was not the problem. My gallbladder was damaged from chemo, but it wasn't the source of my pain. Who needs a gallbladder anyways, right?

Another doctor thought it might be more auto-immune related, which was confirmed by a blood test. He put me on a prescription of Gabapentin, which helped a lot. The pain was still an issue, but it was definitely a lot more under control.

Months passed and the chest pain became increasingly more bearable. I would still get bursts of pain, but I kind of got used to them so they didn't bother me as much. They were pretty much a part of my daily routine. I decided I wanted to once again try to get back into running. Cross country season had already started, and up until this point I was going to practice sometimes to help out with times, stretching, and other random stuff. I also decided at the same time that I was going to get back into Tae Kwon Do. I got my black belt a couple of years before my diagnosis, and absolutely loved the sport. I loved competing, especially sparring, and I was pretty good at it. I took a "hiatus" soon after getting my black belt due to a knee injury, only to have that hiatus extended by cancer. But now that I thought I was getting healthy again, I thought I could just pick up where I left off back when I was actually athletic. Soon enough, I tore my hamstring. In hindsight, I'm not surprised and feel really stupid for trying to do so much so quickly.

I was really frustrated at the number of setbacks preventing me from doing things I used to love. I knew God had reasons for allowing it, but at the time I couldn't figure out why. It was like I would never be that healthy, athletic, fit person I used to be. Now I was just sick, tired, and broken. And it seemed like I would be forever.

One thing keeping me positive was my church family. At the start of my junior year I started leading a small group of sixth grade girls. At first they were a hassle, if you have any idea how talkative and energetic a bunch of middle school girls can be you understand. It didn't take me long to get to know them and love each of them so much. I knew I had to be strong in my faith if I was going to be able to teach them anything about God. So, even though I didn't like what God was allowing in my life at that time with my health, I trusted him and made sure my mind was right.

I went through physical therapy for my injury, and as that was getting better, other things were getting worse. I was getting sick almost every time I ate, and experiencing pain in my side where my stomach is, this seemed to actually set off my chest pain. When my stomach would hurt, my chest would hurt. Soon my chest started hurting more and more when my stomach was not hurting until it was again out of control. I had an endoscopy done and was diagnosed with gastroparesis. The chest pain however, was still unexplainable. The gabapentin didn't seem to be helping anymore, and the pain quickly became debilitating. It was the worst in the morning, making it hard to get out of bed and start the day, so I was missing a lot of school. Half the time when I did go to school I'd have to go back home half way through. Eventually I had to start homebound schooling. Not having to go to school made things easier on my physical health, but my mental health was being challenged. I was feeling very lonely and purposeless. The thing I had to look forward to every week was Wednesday night when I got to see my girls. They restored my sense of purpose every week. I prayed so often that God would help keep me strong so I could be a good role model for them.

Skipping forward to senior year, I was back on top of the chest pain and had it under control once again. I don't know why I live on a roller coaster of chest pain, but apparently I do. And I'm fine with that as long as I always come back up. This school year was special because I got to be an intern for the one person who both saved my life and inspired me to pursue a career in healthcare. Working with Dr. Green was such a blessing because I learned so much not only about how to treat patients, but how to treat people.

Now I am in college, at the University of Georgia. I'm still pursuing a career in healthcare, but have changed from pre-med to public health. I want to get a Master's in Public Health with concentrations in epidemiology and global health and work for the CDC in developing countries to solve and manage disease outbreaks. I'm still interested in cancer, and have been trying to find a position in the university in cancer research. My health is at an all-time high. I still have chest pain quite frequently, but I decided I wasn't going to let that control my life anymore. I deal with it when I have to, and push through what I can. A lot of days I end up on the couch for a few hours with a heating pad and on medication, but I get up the next day, workout, eat healthy, and maximize my health in all aspects that I have control over. I lift weights every day, followed by a run, bike, or swim. I'm currently training for my first triathlon. I've gotten back into sparring, but this time in the form of boxing. I still get sick after eating a lot, but I've learned a lot about what I can and can't eat.

There are two main things that I hope people can get out of my story. The first is that you can only be as healthy as you commit to being. I still struggle with health setbacks every day, but now I refuse to let it stop me from living a healthy life. It would be so easy to skip a morning workout because I was up the night before with chest pain. And it would be so easy to eat unhealthy since I'll probably get sick no matter what I ate, I want to be better than that. I spent too much time feeling sick and tired and broken. I'm not going to let some chest pain hold me back anymore.

The second moral I hope people can learn from my life is that you can do absolutely anything God puts in your path if you surrender your control to Him. Not only did God get me through cancer, he made it enjoyable. Sure, I was painfully sick a lot of the time, but other things totally made up for it. I have had the opportunity to share my testimony with so many people and tell them what God has done in my life. I have had so many people tell me that I inspired them in some way, and that made it all so worth it. I would go through cancer a hundred more times for the opportunity to show people what God can do. He can take what should be the worst times in our lives, and make them the best, most life-changing, heart-warming experiences of our lives. I am so thankful for my cancer journey, because that's how God showed me how wonderful life can be.

Chapter 10

My Fifteen Year Battle with Ovarian Cancer

By Linnea Crouch

September 11, 1967 at 21 years of age, I started working for Delta Air Lines in New York City. It became my special day. I traveled the world, saw things I never dreamed I would see. In between my travels, I became a wife married in Kauai, Hawaii, moved to GA in 1972 a completely different lifestyle than I had ever experienced. It took me a few years to adjust to my new environment but made friends and enjoyed my new way of life. Well, life continued to be interesting and sad at times, a divorce, getting to know myself more, which was a very enlightening experience. Then met my Georgia Southern Gentleman and life elevated to another dimension. We married in 1996 and traveled and then I retired from Delta in 1999. My husband, also a Delta employee retired in 2000, so our plan was to travel more and enjoy the life we had made with each other.

Then in the summer of 2001, I started having pains in my pelvic area that were very intense. I went to my primary doctor as I had tired of the attitude of my gynecologist as sloughing off any complaint I had, as a middle-aged woman of 55. My primary doctor sent me for an ultrasound, which I got a call from him that night to tell me they found a growth on my ovaries. I never had children, several reasons but bottom line; I had heard the risk of ovarian cancer rose for childless women. My primary doctor gave me the name and number of a gynecologist oncologist so that I can make an appointment. I called the next day and the next available appointment was September 11, 2001! It shook me up, I told my husband, and "I don't want to hear any bad news on my special day!"

Well, we know the answer to that one! Not only did our lives change, but also the world changed that day as well. I was scheduled for surgery on Oct.3, 2001, that became my "official diagnosis date" of stage 3C grade 3, serous ovarian carcinoma. Our world changed drastically, new words entered our dialogue. Ports, chemo, Taxol, carboplatin, CT scans, and side effects. Tiredness that caused 4 hour naps, a completely new "lifestyle" much different from the one I experienced in my move to Atlanta so many years ago. Had 18 weeks of the carboplatin and Taxol. Then I was accepted into a clinical trial, which entailed taking Taxol monthly for one year, my last treatment was in 2003. In keeping with our plan to travel, we booked an Alaskan cruise and had a great time. Another part of "our plan" was to keep a positive attitude, enjoy life and do things that we enjoy and try not to let the cancer control our lives. We continued our plan to travel, seeing wonderful sights and experiencing zip lining in Mexico, hot air balloon ride in Sedona, AZ. Other trips and outings that we experienced, as our life was our new normal. We did not let life pass us by, we remain to this day active participants in life. I was very fortunate to be in remission until 2009, Merry Christmas to us…it was back!

2010 started out with surgery in Jan. to remove the growth from my upper abdomen, then a new regimen of chemo in Feb. what they called a 1, 2, 8 a new protocol for chemo. Which in nonprofessional terms was chemo on day 1, day 2 and day 8. It consisted of Taxol, but after a few weeks I developed an allergy so I was introduced to a new medication called Taxotere. A very draining regimen that lasted until June. I was told I would have to be on a monthly chemo for the rest of my life.

After 6 months, I was told I had done so well, CA125 was normal and scans were good that the monthly chemo was discontinued… free again! Of course, during all this (except the 1, 2, 8 period) we had been cruising and traveling, never giving into the treatment. Our treatment was to live life, which my doctor agreed 100 %. One other part of my regimen was to attend Jazzercise classes. I always loved to dance and had started going when I was 40, and attended classes thru most of treatments. The only time I stopped Jazzercise during my 1, 2, 8 protocol, I had to take a leave. I feel that it is so important to have a strong body, because you never know what you have to go through in life, and if your body is strong, it will help get you through "the storm"! My energy level returned to my "old self" and was able to work in the garden and do all my old normal things. I remember one day after planting some flowers and other garden chores breaking down and sobbing. My husband ran over and asked what was wrong. I told him I felt so good, the best I had in such a long time and it was so good to do the things I loved. I will never forget that day. Life went on, traveling and doing fun events.

In late 2013, my CA125 kept rising but scans showed no sign of cancer. By this time in my journey, I had become to feel that the CA125 is just a number that is used as a guide, but not the best tool to judge your "ovarian" health. We continued with our lives and had non-related health bump in the road. We came home from a cruise to a flooded house and had to live in a hotel for 2 months. We were able to go back home on Dec. 24.

2014, started to be a good year, even though my August CA125 showed a count of 732. Well then came October and a count of 1421. Pet scan showed a recurrence. I had ascites, never heard of it. Cancerous fluid starts in the abdomen. Internet did not help my attitude, said usually a 52-week survival rate! I had learned to try a take what you read on the web with a grain of salt. Which is evident since I am now way past 52 weeks. However, it did shake my world! Since there is, no "tumor" to take out you are at the "mercy" of chemo to try to destroy this fluid. The fluid grows and you look like you are pregnant! Well, let me say right up front that the third time has not been a charm. This has been the hardest part of my journey. Jan. 2015 I started on a regimen of Gemzar and Doxil, which I could not tolerate the Gemzar.

In Feb. I had a paracentesis, which I had never heard of, but am now quite familiar with the procedure. They put a tube in your stomach and drain the fluid. The first time I had that done I lost 10 lbs., kind of like liposuction I guess but it's not fat, it's cancer they are taking out of your body. However, it grows and then you need another procedure. Unfortunately, because of all of my surgeries it is difficult for them to do the paracentesis without the guidance of an ultrasound. Let me just say I have lost 40 lbs. from my "drains".

Luckily, I had the extra weight to lose. I told my husband he had better watch out! I was getting down to my "hunting weight" when I was single. Well I do not need to hunt and more. I have a fantastic man who has stood by my side literally. He holds my hand while they put the large needles in my body and holds me when I have a "Moment". This journey could not have been done as sweetly and lovingly without my husband. I am a very fortunate woman to have him in my life and to have survived thus far with this disease. I am still in my battle, and will continue to fight. The fluid has now gone to my lung cavity so I have to have my lungs cavities drained about every 4 weeks. I had to stop going to Jazzercise for a month or so since I had trouble breathing. I was unaware that the fluid made my lungs collapse! That is why I could not breathe. However, had a good drain last week so I've gone back to Jazzercise.

As far as chemo is concerned, I am now chemo resistant so all the chemo that I had in 2014 and part of 2015 was useless. I will not go into all of that year it was very difficult. I now have a doctor that is using an inhibitor (a new type of cancer drug), on me, and my CA125 is below 1,000 for the first time in 2 years. However, scans still show ovarian cancer in the fluid drained from my abdomen and chest. New drugs are being developed every day.

We still plan to travel, not as far, but we are still active in going out and doing fun things with friends and relatives. I still remain positive. Sometimes I will admit it has been difficult but I will not give up. I did not like the attitude of the doctor I went to in 2014 and some of 2015 so I changed doctors. Do not let anyone take

89

away your hope and will to live. You must be your own advocate in your health.

Chapter 11

Mom is Here to Stay

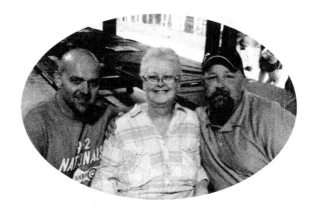

By
John Davis
Stephanie Davis
Brianna Davis

John Davis
(Son of Brenda Davis)

For thirty-nine years the words ovarian cancer never crossed my lips. Unfortunately, the last four years I cannot think of a day that it has not crossed my mind. My mother was diagnosed Stage 3 ovarian cancer in early 2012. I did not know what it was, what it did, or anything else about it, I just knew it was cancer.

I spent the next year and a half watching the women who had cared for me my entire life, suffer unbearably with this depilating disease, but through it all she never quit fighting or give up hope. I felt extremely fortunate to have been able to spend as much time with her as I did, and be able to be by her bedside on a warm morning in June, when she went home to be with the Lord.

Her battle had finally ended, but little did I know mine was just about to begin. I spent the rest of the summer in an angry and depressed state of mind. It wasn't until we walked in the GOCA 5K that Fall, that I started to realize that I wasn't alone. There were other people that had been through the same thing I had been going through.

I started handing out symptom cards and bracelets to women everywhere I went. Slowly but surely, life started to look a little brighter to me, and I began to understand my mother didn't have to die in vain, that it was up to me to keep her memory alive through my life, and the things that I would do to educate and bring awareness to ovarian cancer.

Stephanie Davis
(Daughter-in-law of Brenda Davis)

Brenda Davis, was not just my mother-in-law, she was my mother and a great friend. She was the balance in our family dynamic that most families need and don't have, I was lucky. While most, if not all, my friends couldn't stand their in-laws (especially their mother-in-law) I loved mine, just as much as my own parents. I told everyone that I had the best in-laws and I truly meant it.

Brenda was a woman whom everyone flocked to. She was kind and funny and always there when you needed her. She was beautiful both inside and out. She would never poke into your business, but would be the first one to come to the rescue when you were in need. She would listen and never judge.

One thing I enjoyed about Brenda the most was her voice. I loved to hear her sing. Jason plays the guitar and at family get-togethers and holidays they would pull the guitar out. We would all sit around and just listen. Sometimes I felt bad because I was always the one asking for them to play. I had to pester pretty hard sometimes to get my way. Now I'm glad I did. I think I would give anything to hear Brenda's voice again. Heaven truly gained an amazing Angel when he brought Brenda home three years ago.

Brenda's case was typical of most women that are affected by this disease. She didn't feel well and she was tired all the time. She may have had some of the other symptoms as well because they are common ailments that most women (and men) face daily. Most women including Brenda brush this stuff off as part of getting older. She didn't get concerned or seek out a doctor until she started retaining fluid. Her stomach started getting very large. It looked almost like a pregnancy belly. They ended up draining about 5 liters of fluid off her stomach. Five liters! That is a lot of fluid when you think of how large a 2 liter bottle of coke is. Of course they tested the fluid and found that it was cancer. When Brenda and Terry broke the news to us she did it the same way we did everything….as a family. When we first found out that she had ovarian cancer, we were all shocked. You hear of cancer affecting other people. You hear the odds and know it's a possibility that it could one day affect someone close to you, but you are never prepared to hear it. Even though I was in shock I was hopeful. People battle cancer and win all the time. That's what was going to happen with us. She wouldn't die, she couldn't die. It wasn't possible! We all knew God, had faith in God. She would have surgery. They would remove what they could. They would do Chemo. Everything would be back to "normal".

I don't think our life has ever gotten back to "normal". Now I wonder what "normal" is. Life changed from that point on. It had a different meaning. Life now meant FAMILY more than it ever had before. Some of the early things I remember after we found out was the look on my husband's face. The conversations we had in private. The fear he had of possibly losing his mother. I remember Jason decided to hold off on his music career. He had been in the process of working out the logistics of moving to Nashville. His day job has an office there and he was going to be able to transfer. He had a good band and was playing larger venues. He had a manager and it looked like he was going to be moving up pretty quick.

The day we found out the news he pulled us aside and said he wasn't going anywhere - there was no way that he would be out of state while his Mom was going through this. I remember when we told our daughter. She started crying and the first thing she said was she's not going to see me graduate. Then she looked at me and said she's not going to see Jacob grow up. We both lost it then. We were all close before the news always getting together for

94

Sunday afternoon dinners. But now we were together all the time. Several times through the week and all weekend, every weekend. John did have the opportunity to take Brenda to several of her chemo appointments. I know it meant a lot for him to be there and spend that time with her. They were able to talk, joke and laugh. Through it all, Brenda always stayed positive. She never missed one of Jacobs's soccer games, even when she was wore down from chemo she would come. Even when she was so weak she couldn't walk down to the field she would still come and sit in the van on the hill overlooking the field.

I miss Brenda so much. My heart aches, it aches for my husband, for my kids. They had the most amazing women whom they loved unconditionally taken from them way too soon. They had so many plans. She talked constantly about taking Brianna on a cruise when she graduated. They would get online and look at the different boats, the different destinations. Being sick she was more concerned about the grandkids than she was herself. She worried that Jacob was too young, being 6 years old. She was afraid that he would grow up and he wouldn't remember her. Oh she was so wrong, that little boy remembers her and misses her and talks about her all the time. I look at my husband and he is a different man, he's not the same person he was before. I can tell that something is missing. He doesn't like to talk about it much. He can talk about ovarian cancer and he can talk about his Mom having it but only surface level conversation. Still after 3 years of her being gone, he will break down and cry because it still hurts him so much. And it hurts me because I know there is nothing I can do to make it better.

After Brenda passed we knew that it was going to be extremely difficult on my father-in-law. They had just celebrated their 40th anniversary and they did everything together. Me, John and Jason talked and decided that we needed to make sure we kept him busy. We invited him to dinner after work. It became a ritual for him to stop by after work. Most times he would eat dinner with us, sometimes he would take something to go, and sometimes he would turn up his nose because we were having something he didn't eat. I laugh out loud just thinking about it. We did really enjoy having him come over, I think we all needed to be together to help us heal.

On the weekends; Terry, John, Jason (here on out referred to as the "boys"), and the kids would go to the dirt races. When Terry was in his 20's, he and his brother-in-law (Brenda's brother, Tommy) would race dirt cars. I heard a story once where Brenda drove the race car! She was practicing for the Powder Puff race that was coming up. Her brother Tommy was in the car with her and for everyone who doesn't know….a race car only has one seat. I heard he was hanging on for dear life! I just wish someone would have video tapped it. Unfortunately, the car was broke down when the Powder Puff took place and she didn't get to enter. When I married into the family it was a tradition for the whole family to go to the Shootout at Dixie Motor Speedway in Woodstock every year. We have tons of memories at that race track. I say that to let you know that racing wasn't anything new to the Davis Family.

So for several months, every weekend the "boys" and the kids would go to the dirt races. Different tracks sometimes two races each weekend. It was definitely keeping them all busy and active. One weekend they attended a race at Hartwell Motor Speedway. They were having an event called Pause for a Cause. The race cars were painted up for different causes. The most common being Pink for Breast Cancer Awareness. This really upset the "boys". You always see information, advertising and awareness being displayed for Breast Cancer, but what about Ovarian Cancer? When Brenda found out she had Ovarian Cancer none of us had heard of it let alone knew anything about the symptoms, the side effects, the risks associated with it or the life expectancy. Then they had an idea……..

After the race the "boys" approached me with their idea. They wanted to buy a race car!! Of course my response was "What.... are yawl crazy!?!?!" I thought they were out of their minds. I think if it was my husband asking alone if he could do it, I would have immediately responded with "Ahhh No". But it wasn't just my husband....it was the "boys". I guess there is safety in numbers. I let them finish their proposal to me. They didn't just want to buy a race car, they wanted to buy a race care and paint it up for Ovarian Cancer Awareness. Now they had my attention.

You heard of the movie "We bought a Zoo", well we bought a RACE CAR!! It was decided that John and Jason were going to take turns driving the car. We lettered with Teal Ribbons and Ovarian Cancer Awareness. We were able to go online and find information about ovarian cancer. We made paper pamphlets that had a small story about us with a picture of the race car and then information about ovarian cancer. At the track we would talk to everyone and tell them our story and give them a pamphlet. We just didn't stick to the track either, we made sure to spread word to all of our family, friends and co-workers.

One day a co-worker brought me the Atlanta Journal Constitution. She was aware of what my family was doing and trying to accomplish. Inside was an article on Chris Baxter. Chris's wife, Virginia, was battling Ovarian Cancer. In order bring attention to this disease and to educate everyone in his circle, he had lettered his SUV and Bass Boat for Ovarian Cancer Awareness. This was amazing. Someone else in Georgia was doing the same thing we were. What was even more amazing is when I looked up his information I found that Chris and his wife lived in the same town as us. What a small world!! I was able to message Chris on Facebook and let him know who we were and what we were doing. We wanted to see if we could team up.......join forces so to speak. Through Chris is how we met the group at GOCA.

Now we are on our third year racing and our second year being GOCA partners. Being partnered with GOCA has helped us reach a wider audience than before, when we were doing it on our own. We started out at racing at a couple of tracks to now visiting eight different race tracks. From handing out homemade pamphlets to having pocket sized symptom cards, bracelets and pins. The car looks amazing and draws a crowd everywhere we go. I have women tell me that even though their family member or friend may be racing against us – they secretly pull for us to win. I love when men, women and kids come up to the race car when we stop to get gas or eat on the way to the track. We always love it when the kids get in the car to get their picture taken. It's a great opportunity to share awareness and knowledge. It makes me happy. It makes me feel like Brenda's life wasn't taken in vain. It makes me feel that even though Brenda died another women may live.

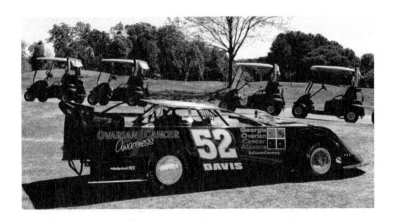

In Memory of Brenda Davis
"Forever Lives in Our Hearts"

Chapter 12

Courage I Never Knew I Had

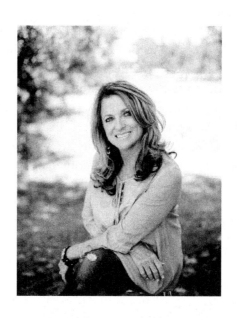

By Sue Durham

"Courage is not the absence of fear, but rather the judgment that something else is more important than fear." Ambrose Redmoon

Sunday July 17th, 2011. My life would take a drastic turn and I would find myself digging deep to find courage I never knew I had. After being taken to the ER I would discover there was a large mass on my right ovary. As soon as I heard the words from the doctor I knew what that meant. There was a very good reason I had been having unusual symptoms in my abdomen.

Fast forward two weeks, August 5th, I was at St. Joseph's Hospital preparing to have the mass removed. Neither my gynecologist nor my oncologist was certain if the tumor was cancerous. My son, now 28, and daughter, now 24, along with a friend were there giving me support. Having them there meant everything, and I knew my children were extremely concerned. During the five plus hour surgery they waited patiently for the doctor to come out and talk. He confirmed the tumor was successfully removed, but that it was cancerous. When I finally woke, one of the first things I noticed was my daughter's face. She had been crying. The tumor was Stage 1 but Grade 3 Clear Cell. Clear Cell tumors are very fast growing, and my oncologist was ready to start chemotherapy treatments as soon as I was able. It would be the most aggressive form of treatment for this kind, a 21 day cycle with treatments on day 1, day 2, and day 8 for the next five months.

The oncologist was optimistic, and his plan was for me to be cancer-free! Of course I would need to stick to the plan and do my part in healing. I was ready to be well again, but I was extremely concerned about the drugs I'd be given and how they would affect my body. The night before my first treatment I was on the phone with the doctor trying to decide if I should or shouldn't do chemo. He sealed it for me when he said, "In a few years if this comes back, would you rather kick yourself for not having treatments or know you did all you could do in the beginning?" So, toward the end of September, with a brave spirit and a nervous smile, I was at the hospital bright and early for that first treatment! I was scared to death, and my sweet nurse knew it. By the third or fourth treatment she had seen a drastic improvement! The port I had in my chest as well as my abdomen was a life safer! If you have to be poked with a needle that many times that little device is a must!

I had attended a couple of very helpful classes hosted by the Ga Ovarian Cancer Alliance, GOCA. This organization helped in so many ways to prepare me for the journey. The classes were uplifting, fun, and educational, and I used every bit of information I could get my hands on to help me through. Learning that one of the chemotherapy drugs would definitely make my hair fall out, I got it cut very short. My hair had always been one of my more proud features, and I wasn't sure how the new look would suite me. But the only thing that truly mattered was becoming cancer free!! When it did start falling out shortly after the first set of treatments it wasn't long before the scarfs and bandanas became the new me. Believe me, it wasn't bad at all. In fact, it was liberating, and not having to do my hair saved a whole lot of time!

With sheer determination, and this new journey I'd begun with God, I just knew I was going to be ok; one way or the other! Over the next several months my faith grew and grew. Most days I'd sit and ponder, thinking about my son, my daughter, all we still had to share together, as well as the possibility of connecting with a special someone with which to share the rest of my life! In addition, my son and daughter-in-law told me I would be blessed with my first grandchild the following March! My heart was overwhelmed with both joy and fear. So I prayed a lot, cried, walked, listened to guided meditations, read, prayed some more. I read several inspiring stories of major cancer survivals and knew I was a fighter too! I attribute much of my recovery to staying home, not working, and focusing on getting well. For anyone reading this and about to go through treatment please try your best to do the same. The bills can wait! Put all undue stress aside, and focus on taking care of you! Let family and friends help when they can, stay as active as possible, eat as healthy as you can, and be diligent about your path to good health! Align yourself with a caring organization like GOCA. They can direct you to women who've been down this road. People who've been here or are still going through treatment can be a great source of comfort.

It takes more than one avenue to treat and beat cancer, and Chemotherapy, as frightening as it can be, it is one very vital treatment. Also, if you've never done meditation now may be the best time to give it a try. There are many forms, and one that really worked for me was guided meditation. Almost every day I would sit quietly and visualize my place of serenity. On the beach listening to waves crash against the shore, and sitting high on a mountain top looking out over the vastness with a cool breeze blowing through the trees. Also, music therapy is used to treat many diseases, and since I've always loved music, I'd put on my earplugs and choose something that connected with my soul. If your mind and body are relaxed and less stressed it has a much better chance to heal itself. Life can always get complicated, but after fighting to be cancer free, the complexities will seem far less important. I pray I never have to go through cancer again, and I pray if you're in that place now, healing is coming your way.

This past August 5th was my 5 year anniversary. Even though cancer is something I never want to have to do again, I am grateful for the experience, as crazy as that may sound! My faith has grown so much, and my spirit shines brighter because of what I've been through. I know where I stand with my God, and even though day to day living can sometimes suck me in, I always seem to rebound, and I try harder each day to remember my blessings. I've always loved nature and the great outdoors, but I believe my experience battling cancer has made me really feel the life in all things. I try hard to be fully present each day, and even though sometimes I struggle more than others, life itself just seems so much more alive!

"You gain strength, courage, and confidence by every experience in which you really stop to look fear in the face. You must do the thing which you think you cannot do." Eleanor Roosevelt.

May God's Grace Be with You!

Chapter 13

Ana's Angels Teal the End

By Heather Eden
(Friend of Ana Virginia Castro Jenkins)

Ana was a loving daughter, sister, cousin, friend and most importantly the mother to two beautiful daughters. Clara and Emilia share the story of their mother's journey through ovarian cancer as a way to honor her memory and help educate others.

On the afternoon of March 2000, Clara called Emilia into her office to share the news that their beloved mother had cancer and that the cancer had metastasized. The very word metastasized, stopped Emilia in her tracks. How could this be that her mother has cancer?

Ana had been sick for many years as she suffered from chronic heartburn, constant abdominal pain, irregular bleeding and abdominal bloating, but the doctors had put her on medication for all these ailments without ever giving the severity any further thought. The doctors gave Ana hormones and suggested that she see a therapist to help her cope with menopause. Ana also underwent surgery for a hiatal hernia that they believed was causing the heartburn. After the operation Ana still did not feel any relief. Clara remembers that the operating doctor told Ana that her ailments were all in her head because the surgery had been a success. Ana was devastated and the girls were heartbroken that no one would listen to their mother. The doctors would not investigate further into the symptoms that Ana was experiencing.

As it turns out all of the "ailments" that Ana suffered from for so many years are the exact symptoms of ovarian cancer. In March of 2000, Ana was diagnosed with Stage 4 Metastatic Ovarian Cancer. Ana fought her battle as hard as she could but lost her battle December 29, 2001.

Ana's cry out for help was never heard. Emilia remembers her tears rolling down her face telling her that she knew something was wrong with her yet no doctor took the appropriate steps to rule out this evil killer. Ana was 54 years old when she died. The bravest, most selfless woman we have ever known. During one of her many hospital stays, Emilia and Clara remember asking Ana if she was scared and her response was that she was not scared for her, she was worried about her beautiful girls. At the time it didn't seem like anything out of the ordinary, she was always worried about her girls. As the years have gone by and the girls have become parents they have realized that Ana's worry was pain, pain in knowing what her daughters were about to have to face, a life without their mother, which has changed Emilia and Clara forever.

Ana's four grandchildren Lucas, Juliana, Adriana and Liliana will never get to meet this amazing and selfless human being. The loss of Ana has been an enormous void that will remain forever. Clara and Emilia believe that the death of their mother could have been prevented had it not gone misdiagnosed for so many years.

In 2006, Emilia married Steve Welchel in Costa Rica surrounded by all of their loved ones. Steve Welchel, co-owner of Marietta Wrecker Service watched his wife's mother, Ana Virginia Castro Jenkins go through her fight against Ovarian Cancer. During a planning session in the fall of 2015, Marietta Wrecker Service decided that one of the goals for 2016 was to give back to the community in a unique way. The Company decided to dedicate a truck in honor of Ana and to help spread awareness throughout the community.

On March 24, 2016, Marietta Wrecker Service (MWS) held a Truck Dedication event that revealed the new Ovarian Cancer Awareness truck. Steve surprised his wife, Emilia Welchel by letting her think that the company was shooting a commercial. During the opening of the ceremony Steve said a few words:

"Thank you for all being with us today as we have this celebration. Today marks a special day for Marietta Wrecker Service. Something that affects all of our lives in one way or another is Cancer. The American Cancer Society estimates that in 2016 more than 22,000 new cases of Ovarian Cancer will be diagnosed and over 14,000 women will die in the US. Mortality rates for Ovarian Cancer have declined only slightly in the 40 years since the "war on Cancer" was declared. Other cancers have shown a much greater reduction in mortality due to the availability of early detection test and improved treatments.

MWS is taking a stance in the fight against Ovarian Cancer. Our hope is that we can raise awareness and make a difference. Ovarian Cancer took the life of someone we love and because of that we wanted to honor her memory in a very special way. On December 29, 2001, my wife and her sister, Clara lost their mother to Ovarian Cancer. Today we dedicate truck 149 in honor of Ana Virginia Castro Jenkins."

The driver of the Ovarian Cancer Awareness truck wears a TEAL uniform every day and gives out information as well as awareness bracelets in an effort to spread awareness and educate people on this silent killer. Every Tuesday is celebrated company wide as TEAL TUESDAY. Everyone on our team has a TEAL TUESDAY uniform. The MWS Facebook page dedicates every Tuesday to Ovarian Cancer Awareness to help educate and spread awareness.

MWS feels so passionately about the cause that they felt they needed to do more and make a bigger impact. The natural thing was to partner with GOCA, Georgia Ovarian Cancer Alliance. Together we can make a bigger difference. MWS wanted to reach a group of people and support the Georgia Ovarian Cancer Alliance (GOCA).

The MWS team and our family feel strongly that education is key, awareness is a MUST!

In loving memory of Ana.

Chapter 14

Lunch & Learn Saved my Life

By Kim Emory

Every survivor has a story and this is mine. Ovarian Cancer crept into my life with illusive persistence. At the time of my diagnosis I had already endured months of pain and anxiety. My symptoms were the classic ovarian cancer symptoms: general abdominal discomfort, bloating, fullness after a meal, nausea, diarrhea, constipation, frequent urination, and unusual fatigue. I also had some other symptoms like indigestion, back pain, and pain with intercourse. When I say I had these symptoms, I had them EVERY single day, some days worst than others, but every day nonetheless.

My relationships were changing and my emotions were in a constant state of turmoil. It is little wonder that this disease is sometimes called the silent killer. I was seeing my PCP at least once or twice a month, and some months as many as three times. Every time I saw, my PCP I would tell her I have a feeling of fullness, and my left side felt as if something was moving. She was giving me everything from anti nausea drugs (promethazine) to drugs for acid reflux, to antibiotics for kidney and urinary tract infections. Once she even put me on a liquid diet saying I had pancreatitis. I was popping Alka Seltzer like they were breath mints; I had long stopped putting them in water and was slipping them under my tongue. Let me not forget to mention all of the BLOOD test and other tests and specialist I was referred to. I had X-Ray's, upper and lower GI's, a colonoscopy and abdominal CT scans. I went to two different GI docs. One GI specialist even had the nerve to tell me I needed to see a psychiatrist because this was all in my head. After I gave him a piece of my mind and a lesson on bedside manner I left his office with no answers.

I had several ER visits one in November of 2005 and one in January 2006 where I was given CT scans of abdomen and drugs for reflux and nausea. I knew something was wrong with me I would leave every doctors visit with no answers but knowing "something is wrong I can feel it." I would spend hours reading online about symptoms, get overwhelmed, and decide I was making a big deal out of nothing. I believe that if I knew about ovarian cancer, the symptoms and the lack of diagnostic testing, I would have been more vigilant and realized that the changes in my body were not "silent" but were there to make me pay attention.

It wasn't until I attended a Lunch & Learn at my job sponsored by the Georgia Ovarian Cancer Alliance, in early 2006, that things started to come together. As I said before I had never heard of ovarian cancer. I listened to the speaker and afterwards took a symptom and risk card, returned to my desk put the card in my desk drawer, and continued to get sicker. One day I came to work and opened my desk, mind you I did this everyday but that day was like the first time I had ever opened my desk, and the symptom card from GOCA glowed. I looked at the card, decided to read the symptoms, and started to check off the symptoms I had, abdominal pain - check, bloating - check, frequent urination - check, feeling of fullness after a meal - check, and nausea - check. I had all of the symptoms on that card except for one, vaginal bleeding. I immediately called my PCP, asked if I could come in and see her, and that I had a card I wanted her to see. My husband and I got to her office and I handed her the card, it was as if a light bulb came on. She called her nurse and the referral coordinator in her office and told them to get me an immediate appointment that day for a PET scan. She then told me she feared I had Ovarian Cancer. My husband and I left her office dazed. After a year and a half of back and forth, many test, and seeing a few specialists I finally had something that made sense.

My PCP and I both, through divine intervention, found the worlds best (in my opinion) Gynecologic Oncologists. After looking at my scans, they set me up for surgery immediately. My ovarian cancer surgery and diagnosis came three days after my dear beloved Auntie Nora had suddenly passed away. She was my Libra sister - I was born two days after her birthday on Oct. 12. Since I had lost my parents, my mother in 1995 and my father in 1999, I could always count on her for support and advice. She always held a very special place in my heart. Devastated by her death I contemplated putting off the surgery until after her funeral, but on the advice of my doctor, trusted family members and friends I decided to have the surgery. So on March 17, 2006 my left ovary, fallopian tube, omentum and appendix were removed. When I woke up from surgery, surrounded by my husband, three of my cousins, a very dear friend and my doctor, the pain in their eyes was so evident. The doctor had sent my tumor to pathology, and based on preliminary pathology he was already pretty sure of it was ovarian cancer. My God I was face-to-face with ovarian cancer!

I had Stage IIc Ovarian Cancer; specifically I was diagnosed with a rare germ cell tumor for my age (39) called Endodermal Yolk Sac. Cancer is like Jason from the Friday the 13th movies. It is big and scary and you don't really know how you are going to deal with a big ugly monster like that until you stare it in the face, and here I was staring this Friday the 13th like monster in the face. Do you run and hide and hope that it won't get you? Or do you stand and fight and kick its ass? I chose to fight and kick its ass! Everything happened to me pretty quickly, from surgery to diagnosis to chemo in less than a month, Mar. 17th-surgery, Mar. 24th-final diagnosis, Apr. 7th-chemo. Somewhere between surgery and chemo I had another "minor" surgery to put the port in. I hated seeing that thing every day and it hurt like hell for them to access it. It looked like a little bottle cap underneath my skin. I totally recommend getting a port, but I was so grateful when it was removed. My surgeon wanted to know if I wanted to keep it. Some people do as a reminder. No way. Thanks for the memories, but throw that thing away. I have enough memories/scars of all I went through.

The next four months were tough for me and everybody around me. There is nothing good I can say about chemotherapy. It sucked! My chemotherapy regime was very aggressive and I needed all the help I could get. So, my mother-in-law and 80-year-old aunt came from Cleveland, Ohio and Augusta, Georgia to stay with Erik, and me and help out for a while. I had three twenty-one day cycles, a total of sixty-two days of the worst chemo drugs imaginable (Etopiside, Bleomycin and Cisplatin). I was very sick from the chemotherapy. That napalm they give you caused all of my hair to fall out. There were times when I couldn't eat, and when I was so fatigued from chemo/napalm, but couldn't sleep because of the steroids they gave me to "help".

I sometimes ask myself the question, "Why?" Not so much why I was the one to get cancer, but rather, why am I the one who survived; the one who got a second chance? The only answer I can find is that we are all in this world for a reason. I think I am here to make some laugh and to make some cry. I would love to think that I am here to make some see that life is too short to be wasted and too precious to be ignored. Throughout this experience I have realized my own strengths. I fought this disease with everything I had and even though I lost things doing it: a year of my life, my hair (I know it's just hair but wait until you lose it, or as mine did fall out in patches), friendships and the ability to have children. However, I have gained some things that are far more valuable, a renewed faith and a passion for life. I have gone through something only some ever will. Having cancer does not mean your life is over. Rather, it means it has just begun. Mine has anyway. I wish to make others see this too. Life after cancer is possible. It is possible to have this disease, fight it, and move on.

Ten years later it's mind-boggling how far removed from my ovarian cancer diagnosis I am, but yet how close I remain. I still can't believe that was me, chemo bound, bald and scared out of my mind. I don't ever want to lose my connection with ovarian cancer, I hate it...but I love who I've become because of it. There are still those Moments that I get that sinking feeling. Even as I write this, my mind is racing and the tears are flowing...I'm okay now, yet there was a real chance I wouldn't be. Having a disease like ovarian cancer has provided me an opportunity to evaluate my life. It has also afforded me an opportunity to think about my relationship with God. I grew-up a Southern Baptist, but being told you have ovarian cancer put new meaning into those prayers that can sometimes become customary. Someone once asked me to explain to them how I could believe in God. As I sat thinking I was like, hey that's not something I can do. If you're looking for the logic in my belief, it's not there, but I do know that God cares for me and that He has a good place awaiting me when it's my time to go. I credit God, my medical caregivers, my family members and my own stubbornness for my survival of this disease. I truly believe that this cancer journey/war has been a blessing. My biggest blessing/supporter has been my husband of twenty years, Erik. He has been with me every step of the way from connecting my IVs, driving me here and there, and pushing me at times when I had no will. All of this has not been without a few choice words from both of us, but no one has been privileged to have more love than I have.

I am now an expert in something I never wanted to be an expert in, ovarian cancer. I wish I could say that I didn't know anyone else who's been diagnosed with this disease, but that is not the case. I've often contemplated what can I do to help others prevent and survive ovarian cancer. There seems to be no rhyme or reason to this insidious disease. Even so, I have lots of information and experiences to share with you about it. Though I am incredibly sorry that more women have been diagnosed, I am glad that I can provide some help and support based on my own experience. In honor of those women I know who didn't make it, and as a survivor myself, I have a responsibility to make the best use of my life... to help as many women/men as I can ... to live strong with or without ovarian cancer. For survivorship to be meaningful to me it requires a certain level of lasting responsibility.

My world has become broader. I've had the pleasure of meeting ovarian cancer survivors from around the country. I've done television interviews, wrote newspaper and magazine articles, interviewed for a pod cast, and done numerous health fairs. I continue to sit on the Board of Directors of the Georgia Ovarian Cancer Alliance (GOCA) currently as president. I participated in the GOCA's Survivors walk, GOCA's Survivors Teaching Students® - Saving Women's Lives, GOCA's annual "Shaken, Not Stirred" galas and the Ovarian Cancer Research Fund Alliance conferences and advocacy days held in Washington D.C. I got to be part of the world in a bigger way than I have before. The woman who started this race is definitely not the same woman who is finishing it.

For the past several weeks, I thought about writing my story for this book with a combination of reverence, anxiety, grief, delight, and liberation. Sounds crazy, huh? Well welcome to my "new normal" the life of a cancer survivor. When you are a cancer survivor, you have this date engraved in your memory like your birthday, wedding day, or September 11, the day Prince died. You'll never forget where you were or what you were doing when you heard the words, "You have cancer." For me that date is March 17, 2006, a kind of new birthday. My life as I knew it would never be the same again, no matter the outcome. I never planned on becoming an ovarian cancer survivor because, like most people, I never planned on having ovarian cancer. When you're a young woman, getting on with your life, cancer let alone ovarian cancer, is the last thing on your mind.

Although this cancer journey has been long and some times frightening, along the way I have met many amazing women who I am proud to call sister-friends. We are all at different stages of our cancer journeys, but united in our desire to be there for each other through this rollercoaster ride our lives have now become. From the time I first heard the words "you have cancer", I was surrounded with love and support. Support I am still humbled by today. From prayers, meals, cards, to those who would sit quietly with me in the infusion center, and I have loved it all.

What helps me find meaning in all of this is a deep desire to give something back, to help others with a diagnosis of cancer. I have a story that needs to be shared so that others will not feel alone in their fight against cancer. I look to the future and vow to make the best life I can for myself and those I care about and in the process to hopefully touch the lives of others with some of the compassion and love I was given. The more I do, the more I want to do.

Dictionary.com defines survivor as a person who continues to function or prosper in spite of opposition, hardship, or setbacks. For some cancer patients the word survivor does not do justice to the power they felt fighting cancer. They want words that evoke the newfound power they attained since being diagnosed. They want words like slayer, warrior or fighter. Also some in the cancer community say survivor does not pay homage to the ones who succumbed to cancer. I have a hard time understanding why it is a big deal for some. In my opinion I am living after fighting this deadly beast so I am surviving. So for me, the term survivor is more than just a catchphrase; it›s a call to action, a way to establish some sense of power in a situation where losing control can happen very quickly. So call me what you want warrior, fighter, slayer, princess, queen or bitch. But what I am truly is a person who continues to function or prosper in spite of opposition, hardship, or setbacks. A true SURVIVOR...yeah that's me!

After the fog cleared and I began adjusting to my new life-- as an ovarian cancer survivor --in my opinion you are always a survivor. I began to look for ways to deal with the new me. Advocacy has given me a tool to continue fighting this disease, not only for me but also for those who are fighting, those who have lost their battles and women who don't know that they may be at risk. Speaking out works - by getting involved, breast cancer survivors have increased funding for breast cancer that has led to new treatments and tests that are saving more lives than ever before. We in the ovarian cancer community are and need to continue doing the same for ovarian cancer. As advocates for ovarian cancer we are educating women about ovarian cancer, changing public policy, and making a difference! Through this thing called ovarian cancer I have had the opportunity to meet and become friends with some of the most courageous and impressive women on this earth. If not you...then who! Take action y'all!!!

Today I am thankful for a lot of things, friends and family, To all the people who have helped me through this, whether you realized it or not, thank you.

So why do I want to share my story? I share my story because I have joined the sisterhood of ovarian cancer survivors. I share my story because I like so many other women who have endured the shock of having cancer, battling cancer with the surgeries and chemotherapy treatments and the continual fear of cancer recurring, l have a story to tell. I share my story so that women of all ages are reminded of how important it is to always be aware of the very subtle warning signs of ovarian cancer. I share my story in the hope that you do experience unusual symptoms (bloating, pelvic, or abdominal pain, difficulty eating, feeling full quickly, and feeling a frequent or urgent need to urinate); you will seek medical attention even though you might be fearful of the results. I share my story so that we as a community can become better educated regarding the facts and correct treatments so that unnecessary risks are avoided. I share my story in the hope that these, actions offer you the opportunity of dramatically improving your chances for survival.

I share my story because after being diagnosed with ovarian cancer and enduring three twenty-one day rounds of chemotherapy (three different drugs everyday), which I completed on July 11, 2006, I am cancer-free. I share my story so you can see that the check-ups every three to six months are still nerve-wracking. I share my story because it is comforting to know that I am being followed very closely. I share my story so that you will know that throughout this experience, there were so many things in my life that helped me to remain strong and positive; support from friends, family, co-workers, doctors, nurses, and a husband who never left my side were the most significant.

I share my story so that people will know that I have gained so much. I share my story because I am excited about the new research in ovarian cancer, which is leading us towards more effective screening tools and better treatment. I share my story because of the pain and sadness I have felt when I hear about sisters who have lost their battle against this disease. I share my story because I have been overcome by fear and anxiety as I await results of blood work every six months, wondering if my cancer has come back. I share my story because as horrible as this disease is, I wouldn't trade anything for this journey. (I know that sounds cliché coming from a survivor, but it is true.) I share my story because I will continue to fight this monster called ovarian cancer and share my story so maybe someone else will have a chance of an early diagnosis, which will lead to a very long remission. I share my story because I am still here!

Chapter 15

Ovarian Cancer
"This is the Day the Lord has made,
I will rejoice and be glad in it!"
Psalms 118:24

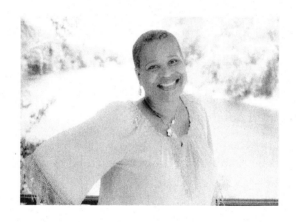

By
Gailtricia Brenlyn Thomas Fogg
Tracy Fogg
Brenton Fogg
Tracy "Aparicio" Fogg, II
Robin Tutt Mole
Carol Spain

My Daily Declaration

This is the Day the Lord has made, I will rejoice and be glad in it! Psalms 118: 24

An Attitude of Gratitude

Personally, I have had a few struggles in my life that taught me to hold on to an attitude of gratitude and be thankful even in the struggles:

I have learned to be thankful for life, when our oldest son, Tracy "Aparicio" Fogg, II, then age eight was run over by a car and not expected to live because his skull was separated like a perfectly cracked egg all the way around and his brain was knocked offline.

Because he had to relearn everything all over again and it took several years to do this, I have learned to be thankful for things that most people do not think about, like...

I learned to be thankful for a blink, when he blinked his eyes for the first time after the accident;

I learned to be thankful for a sneeze, a nod, the ability to sit up without falling over, the words, mama, dada, a smile, etc.;

I learned to be thankful for when my husband told the doctors in the pediatric intensive care unit to get ready for the biggest miracle that they have ever seen in the Children's Hospital and our son was named the first Miracle Child for the Children's Miracle Network for the Medical Center of Central Georgia.

I learned to be thankful for my 93-year-old mother, when we had to take care of her in my home, when she got dementia. She taught me to see things her way, like when she was watching a basketball game on television and said, "Tricia, look at those boys playing basketball in your back yard" and I said, "Yes ma'am, I see them, they are having fun!"

...and for her ability to make me laugh like when I was bald and she looked up at me and said, "Tricia, you don't have a bit of hair on your head." I told her it was the new style and she responded, "I'm not sure if I like that style."

I was also thankful that even though sometimes my mother did not remember her only child's name, she remembered the words to the song that we sang each morning, "Rise, Shine and Give God glory."

I was even thankful that because of the dementia, she didn't know that her "little girl" was battling ovarian cancer.

I am also thankful that God gives us the wonderful gift of memories after she passed away on January 1, 2013. There is not a day that goes by that I do not think about her.

And, I learned to be thankful for each and every Moment of the day when I was diagnosed with one of the biggest health challenges a person could face.

I am a survivor of ovarian cancer stage 3C. It is no secret that cancer turns your life upside down in an instant. With so much uncertainty and stress, some would ask, how is it possible to have an attitude of gratitude? Well it turns out that adversity can make you more thankful, as you recognize the value of the people and experiences that have enriched your life.

Life Changing Moment

One life changing Moment for me began when I started to have pelvic pain. I thought that I had a bladder infection, but when medicines did not help, I told my doctor that he had to look inside of me to see what was going on. I immediately had scans to find out that I had a significant size mass on the one ovary that I had left, I was told that I had to have surgery to remove the ovary and that I either had Endometriosis or Ovarian Cancer but I would not know until after the surgery. Dr. Alan Gordon explained to me what would happen in each case. When telling me about the chemotherapy if it were cancer, he told me that I would lose my hair and then he paused. "I said ok and then what?" He told me that some people were devastated when they found out that they may lose their hair. My response was, "I could care less about losing my hair, I just do not want to lose my life."

On December 14, 2011, I woke up from surgery to find out that my life would be changed by Ovarian Cancer Stage 3C.

Journal entry for December 23, 2011.

Saying thank you to my family and friends for your prayers before, during and even now after my surgery! The prayers of the righteous avail much! Please continue to pray for me on this journey! Just know that I am fine as we serve a Mighty God who is God over Everything!! This was no surprise to Him and I know he holds me in His hands! Whatever my lot, Thou has taught me to say, It is well with my soul! All for His glory!!!! By His stripes we were healed!!!!

Thank God for Pain.

Now most of us do not like change, not even in the slightest way but some change cannot be avoided and this was one of them.

I must pause here to say that this is when "I was thankful to God for my pain because this "silent killer" was trying to do just what its "nickname" implies... Always pay attention to your pain, it is usually trying to tell you something.

The pelvic pain that I was having was persistent and extremely uncomfortable. I knew that something was wrong. This was foreign to my normal feelings. I now realize it to be a symptom of ovarian cancer.

Priorities

On the last day in the hospital after my surgery, Dr. Gordon told me to go home and enjoy Christmas and that he would see me back on January 9, 2012. I informed him that I could not see him on that date but I could see him on the following Monday. Of course, he wanted to know why. I told him that I was a teacher, in my 27th year of teaching and that I would be retiring in three years. I informed him that I had a plan that I would have another Master's Degree in Professional Counseling by the time I retired and that this was to be my second career. I also informed him that I was a student at Liberty University and only had 2 classes left, one being a weeklong intensive class and an internship. The weeklong intensive class began on January 9, 2012. I had to be there because I was not putting my life on hold because of cancer. I wanted to be finished with everything by the end of the summer of 2012. He informed me that I could not drive to Virginia and I reminded him that I had a husband who was sitting right beside me who told him, "Dr. Gordon, there is nothing you can say that will stop her, I will drive her." Dr. Gordon then said, "Okay, I will see you on the following Monday."

I went to my intensive at Liberty and while I was there, the head chaplain of The Medical Center of Central Georgia, Sean Beck came to my classroom to recruit interns for the pastoral care department.

Internships were hard to find and I was elated to learn that there was an intern opportunity in my city and that he had come to my class all the way from Macon Georgia to recruit. I took the brochure, introduced myself and prayed that my interview would be good enough. There were 40 applicants and 6 openings. God graced me with the opportunity of landing an internship at the Medical Center of Central Georgia.

Journal Entry for January 25, 2012.

I am convinced and sure that He who began a good work in me will continue until the day of Jesus Christ, developing and perfecting and bringing it to full completion in me. Philippians 1:6

Jesus bore your sicknesses and carried your diseases at the same time and in the same manner that He bore your sins. When you allow the incorruptible seed to go into your heart, it will produce the crop you desire... Every time!

Receive the Word of God. The power and blessing you receive from it will be according to how you hear it. Receive it as God talking to you, as the Word of the living God and the authority in your life!

Chemotherapy

I went to my follow-up appointment with Dr. Gordon and we talked about chemotherapy. I had too many choices. At this time, I needed God to speak to me about chemotherapy but, I could not seem to hear from Him. I did not say that He wasn't speaking, I just could not hear for some reason. I had expected that my doctor was going to just tell me exactly what to do and I would do it, however he gave me three choices: Choice one was to have chemo in my port in my chest. Choice two was to have chemo in my port in my chest and intraperitoneal chemo in my abdomen.

Choice three was to have chemo in my port in my chest and to try a clinical trial with avastin, a drug I would have to take for the rest of my life.

I was at a lost. I did not know which road to take. I thought that he would just tell me what to do which would have been much easier.

I continued to pray and ask God for wisdom. He gave me the right question to ask the doctors. Yes, I did say doctors because I had acquired a second opinion from a doctor in Atlanta. I asked the doctors, "If I were your daughter which choice would you want her to take?" They both said the same thing. The doctor here in Macon, Dr. Gordon said, "I would want you to do IP chemo because the remission time is longer and the survival rate is higher. However, 60% of my patients do not complete their chemo like that because of pain and complications and have to go back to just getting chemo in the port in their chest. Intraperitoneal chemotherapy is putting 2 liters of fluid in your stomach and then turning for two hours from your right side to your back to your left side and visa versa." Its nickname is "Shake and Bake"

The doctor in Atlanta, Dr. Hines basically told me the same thing. He said, "I don't want to discourage you from the IP but two-thirds of my patients do not complete the chemo this way due to pain and complications." It was then that I made up my mind. I told Dr. Hines, "Two thirds of your patients do not complete IP chemo but one third do and I am going to be in the one-third who do complete the IP chemo and I am going to complete it without pain or complications." I came back to Macon and told Dr. Gordon that I had made up my mind. I told him that "60% of his patients did not complete IP chemo but 40% did and that I was going to be among the 40% and that I was going to complete it without pain and complications." He smiled.

Journal Entry for February 10, 2012 .

Ok, so I go to surgery to get ports put in for chemo... that goes well... Then, oh my, a nosebleed for two whole hours... Back to surgery again to cauterize the vessel... Now I have more restrictions from that surgery than the first one! Wow what a wonderful Wednesday it was... Seriously because I'm alive! It could have been worse and I know that Isaiah 40:29,31 says: You give power to me when I am faint and weary. In my weakness, you increase strength in me, I wait for you (expect, look for, and hope in You) and You Renew my strength and power. I will lift up with wings of strength and rise as an eagle. I shall run and not be weary, I shall walk and not faint or become tired.

Decisions

Well, I had several things to think about. First, my youngest son, Brenton Traquez Fogg, was graduating from college with honors on May 9, 2012, and I had to plan chemo around his graduation so that I would be sure to have plenty of energy so that I could celebrate heartily for this awesome accomplishment in his life. On May 17th I was having my first meeting about my internship. I had a lot going on. My life was going on and I was thankful!

I went on to find out that my chemotherapy would consist of 18 times which included intraperitoneal (IP) chemotherapy, which as I stated earlier, was putting 2 liters of fluid in my belly and my turning for 2 hours from my right side to my back to my left side back to my abdomen and so forth.

My chemo regimen was as follows: Monday, I had the chemo taxol, in the port in my chest; Tuesday, I had the chemo cisplatin, in my abdomen and the following Monday, taxol in my abdomen again. I then had two weeks off and it would start all over again.

During the first week, I was usually alright after the first two days, probably due to the steroids that I received intravenously, but it was on the third day that I began to experience weakness and fatigue. I also would have altered taste buds and did not really want to eat because everything tasted like paper. I had to find the one thing that I could somewhat tolerate; it was pineapples.

I had to go back to the doctor every Friday in order to get blood work done.

New Friends

After posting on Facebook about my new diagnosis, a friend, Jenise Gibson that I had gone to church with growing up inboxed me and asked for my number. I sent it to her and she called. She informed me that her 21-year-old daughter had passed away from ovarian cancer and that she had gotten involved with spreading awareness at different events sponsored by GOCA, the Georgia Ovarian Cancer Awareness. She told me that there were two girls that I needed to meet. She had already inboxed them and told them about me. She gave me their telephone numbers and I did not hesitate to call. These two lovely women were ovarian cancer survivors also. When I called Benita Osbey and Kimberly Emory, they were so patient and willing to talk to me for as long as I needed. I called them often and asked what seemed like a thousand questions, many of them more than once. They were always willing to walk with me, helping me in any way possible.

Wig Party

Dr. Gordon had told me that after my second Chemo, my hair would probably begin to fall out. My friends had given me a wig party.

Journal Entry for March 4, 2012.

Friends are God's ways of taking care of us! I have the greatest friends...they surprised me with a "wig" party! It was so much fun... Kinda like little girls playing dress-up ! Thank you guys so much for being here for me! I love you all!

A Birthday Present

What a birthday present! My birthday is March 22nd and I was so grateful to be alive so that I could attend our son, Brenton's college Honors Convocation! God is so good to me!

Journal entry for March 22, 2012.

So proud to be at The Fort Valley State University's Sixty-First Annual Honors Convocation where our son Brenton Traquez Fogg is participating for the fourth year in a row! Not only is he receiving an award for High Academic Achievement but is also being recognized for being included in the Thirty Fifth Edition of the National Dean's List, nominated for membership in Alpha Kappa Mu Honor Society, receiving Departmental Honors as well as The Fort Valley Alumni Award! We are so very proud of you son and how God is shaping your life! I am so grateful to be alive to share this Moment with you! The Best Birthday Ever!

Prayer

I strongly believe in the power of prayer so I asked everyone "When you think of Gailtricia pray these three things: No pain, no complications and no disease left in her body!" I later added, "No low energy".

A New Hairdo

Journal entry for March 27, 2012.

Thank you Lord for this second day of round two with no pain no complications, no disease in my body ever... Now I'm about to get a new hairdo!

I melt in your peace, it's overwhelming!

At this point, I had plenty of wigs to wear. However, it was during the week of the second round when I went to the mirror to comb my hair for church and realized that it was coming out. I told my husband and I made a joke and said, "I guess I won't be primping in the mirror in the restroom at church today!" He smiled.

It was in two days that I called my husband and my sons into the bathroom and said, "Ok guys, we are about to have a hair cutting party!" My husband got out his clippers and began to shave my head. I had to have fun with it so he shaved it in all kinds of shapes at first. I even took a picture with a "Buckwheat curl". We made it a family fun event. After my husband cut it all off, my sons said, "Mom, you look good bald." I looked in the mirror, put on some lipstick and said, "I don't look half bad at all." Brenton is a photographer so he wanted to take all kinds of pictures and he did. We had a blast!

Special Moments

Journal entry for May 8.

I am such a proud Mom! Congratulations to our son Brenton who is graduating tomorrow from " The Fort Valley State College" in just a few hours! He is graduating MAGNA CUM LAUDE! Thank you Lord!

My youngest son, Brenton was about to be a college graduate and I was so grateful to be alive so that I could attend graduation. I was also grateful that I could attend and not be weak or sick. We gave him a huge graduation cookout and had over 90 people to attend. It was totally awesome and for me…prayers answered! I was alive to experience it! What a joy!

Journal entry for May 12, 2012.

I had an awesome Mother's Day! Words cannot begin to express how I felt when my son Brenton, who by the way was born on Mother's Day, and was leading worship, pulled me off the worship team to the front of the stage and told everyone what a strong woman I was and how much he loved me and wanted to give me back everything I had done for him… What a blessing! It took me a while to get it together after that but I feel so loved! Thank you God for two wonderful children and an awesome husband that I am here with and able to enjoy!

This was an exceptional Mother's Day gift for me. First of all, Brenton's birthday was May 13, 1990 and on this day in 1990, it was Mother's Day. He was my Mother's Day gift. Now years later, he is telling me that I am his gift…Look at God!

A Bump in the Road

Journal entry for May 20, 2012.

Ok, so I guess if I just wanted a night away from home, I should have booked the Ritz Carlton rather than the Medical Center of Central Georgia… Oh well, home now and last nights sleep was well in MY bed … Chest pains subsided, magnesium level back to normal and no blood clots Thanks to EVERYONE for your prayers! …My God is Awesome!

Internship

Internship began and the blessing is that the floors that I was responsible for counseling with and ministering to were the "cancer floor" and "women's health" floor. What an awesome opportunity when I would walk into a cancer patient's room with my bald head and the patient would ask, "Are you going through chemo or is that hairdo fashion?" I would answer, "Actually, it is both." I then had a great opportunity to share and patients would open up and share their feelings as well. It's much easier to share when someone has walked a mile in your shoes. This was such a blessing to me. I had no idea what God had in store for my future!

This Too Shall Pass

Journal entry for May 29, 2012.

Getting closer... On my way to my fifth round. After Monday only one more left, Whoo hoo! God has really blessed me to get through this with No pain No complications and No disease and I'm forever grateful! Keep praying that prayer for me... NO DISEASE IN MY BODY EVER AGAIN !!!

"He has great plans for me!"
Jeremiah 29:11

Journal entry for May 30, 2012.

Day 2 of round 5 begins today! Doctor's visit was awesome on yesterday... Numbers looked great! My God is awesome He can move mountains, keep me in the valley, hide me from the rain...

FINAL TRIPS

Journal entry for June 25,2012.

Well, this is one trip I don't mind taking. This is my LAST trip to the infusion center... My last chemo treatment! This has been a journey that I wish for no one but if one must go on it, just don't go without God! He has been so good to me! He has given me exactly what I needed to make it! He put the right people in place to pray and just in place for whatever I needed and I thank Him for that! Thanks to EVERYONE for your prayers and please keep praying! We serve an awesome God who is able to do everything

Journal entry for August 28,2012.

On my way to the hospital and this is another trip I don't mind taking... Today I am getting the ports removed from my belly and my chest because I DON'T NEED THEM ANYMORE! This has been quite a journey but My God had been right by my side the whole way... Y'all, He is so good, please taste and see... There is nothing too hard for Him... Just believe! How Great is our God!!! Thanks to my awesome husband and boys, my extended family and EVERYONE who believed with me and are still believing... From the bottom of my heart, I Love You!

LIVING

I decided that just because I was diagnosed with cancer, that cancer did not define my identity. I believe in having a positive spirit because even research shows that this is more than half of the battle. I tried to recognize something to be thankful for as many times in the day as possible.

I had to make choices, not only about chemotherapy---as a matter of fact choices about the cancer itself--- was not the most important choice I had to make. The most important choice I had to make was "how I was going to "live" my life. Yes "live "my life!

I am naturally an optimistic person and I always try to find the good in things. You may ask, "Where is the good in cancer?" This is not what I mean. What I mean is that I had to find the good in every Moment of every day. It was either this or I have a pity party and die, not literally, although this could have happened, but die while I was living. Well, there's not much fun in that so I decided to "Live"

During my IP chemo, I had to wear a gown because I had to lie down when receiving the chemo. Well, I am a little bit fashionable so each time I went to chemo, my nurses would say something about my jewelry and my matching gown. I mention this not to brag about being fashionable, I mention this because it was part of my "living". One thing I have learned is that you must do what makes you feel special, even in the midst of personal adversity!

HUMOR

Also, as I mentioned before, I had to turn for 2 hours, every 15 minutes from my right side to my back to my left side to my back and so forth. So even though, Gail, my nurse would be there to tell me the time, I would set the alarm on my phone for every 15 min. to play songs like "Turn the Beat Around" by Gloria Estefan or Turn, Turn, Turn by the Birds...I added humor to my chemo experience. Proverbs 17:22 even tells us that a cheerful heart is good medicine but a crushed spirit dries up the bones. Well, I did not want my bones dried up, so I decided to keep a cheerful heart while trusting God.

"SUPER GOOD AND GETTING BETTER"

So when people ask me how am I today, "My answer is usually "Super Good and Getting Better!" "Do I have residual from the chemo? Sure I do. As much as I love to wear heels, the neuropathy in my feet says, "Nope you can't wear those," so I have to find some cute flats or wedges to wear. (It's not the end of the world) And yes, sometimes my joints ache, but you know what, "I am alive to feel all of that" and that is worth me praising God and being Thankful for."

A DIFFERENT VIEW

When going through life and death situations, you begin to view the world through very different lenses. Things that used to be important are no longer on your priority list. Things that used to upset you, are really trivial. Forgiveness even comes easier. These are positive changes that take place inside of you. Every Moment counts and "the small stuff we used to sweat" is looked upon as wasted time. You become grateful for the simple things. "I DON'T SWEAT THE SMALL OR THE BIG STUFF!'

The greatest commandment that God gave us is to Love the Lord your God with all your heart, with all your soul and with all your mind and the second is like unto it, Love your neighbor as yourself.

Love is an action word and I am so glad that I had people around me who loved me and were there carrying me when I was weak. I did not have to go it alone.

The greatest action of love was done by my husband, Tracy and my sons, Aparicio and Brenton who are unsung heroes in that, not only were they taking care of me but also my 93-year-old mother who could not do for herself because of dementia. They took over my duties after I got sick and did an awesome job of loving on her and me.

I believe that Hope is first and foremost found in God. I am grateful that He has given people wisdom so that we can also find Hope in research, new treatments, new drugs, new procedures, and in people like doctors, nurses, health care administrators, counselors, educators, pastors and of course those closest to us, our caretakers, families and friends.

So I encourage others, in the midst of even a dreadful disease like cancer to find hope and "live" by Loving God and people, "living" life and enjoying everyday! And then, "Don't forget to pay it forward!"

A LOOK INTO THE FUTURE

While in the infusion center receiving chemotherapy, I said to Jill Hancock, the head nurse, "You guys need a chaplain just for this area and it needs to be me!" She replied, "You are so right, Gailtricia, it would be wonderful and you would be perfect for the job!"

At the end of my internship, I told my supervisor, Sean Beck, "In three years, I'll be back so that I can do my residency here and work on my hours for licensure for this professional counseling degree. I'm sure that God will open the door and it will be perfect because I will have retired from the school system."

I retired from teaching June 1, 2015 and I began my journey as a resident chaplain on August 31, 2015. Part of my duties include serving as chaplain to the Infusion Center! As William Cowper wrote, "My God works in mysterious ways, His wonders to perform"

"You do not realize now what I am doing, but later you will understand." John 13:7

ACKNOWLEDGEMENTS

I am thankful to God for the loves of my life; my wonderful husband, Tracy and my two sons Aparicio and Brenton who were always there and give me hope even to this day.

My best friend, Vanessa Harvey and my sisters Robin Mole and Michelle Drew who sometimes slept at the foot of my bed. My cousin, Katherine Campbell who is like a mother to me who prayed with me and for me constantly, my Goddaughter, Simone who is a nurse and made sure that I had royal treatment while in the hospital, my Godsister, Carol who helped me so many times with my mother who lived with us while battling dementia and so many others who brought food and gave support.

I appreciate my dear friend and soon to be family member, Janice "Iamfitness" Shepherd, the Zumba Queen, who orchestrated and lead an awesome Zumba fundraiser for me.

My doctors, Dr. Alan Gordon, Dr. Aubrey Harper and Dr. F. Kevin Young were totally awesome and still are today!

A special shout out to my home run hitters, my nurses who were with me at the infusion center: Jill Hancock, my personal nurse Gail Williams, Jennifer Beck, Cindy Bohannen, Carmen Davey, Tonya Greene, Jerald Jewell, Tonya McClain, Shannon Smith and Lynn Watson.

My dear friend, Benita Osbey who often called me her twin when I was bald and answered my every call when I needed someone to talk to. RIP Soror Benita.

My guardian angel, Rheba Drye, a breast cancer survivor, who was with me at 17 out of 18 of my infusions. RIP Mama Rheba.

My sweet angel, my mother, Mattie Julia Jackson Thomas who helped me smile through this journey. RIP Mama

Tracy Fogg
(Husband of Gailtricia Fogg)

Is it cancerous or not? The anticipation was nerve racking. This was the feeling I had on Dec. 14ᵗʰ 2011 as we waited on the doctor to come tell us the results. The scene, not in a movie, but with my wife lying in her hospital bed in the Medical Center of Central Ga. just after having surgery to remove a mass on her ovary and waiting on the results. Just a few days before, I was with her as she was told of the potential diagnosis of a mass found on tests ran to seek answers to her constant pain.

With Tricia at the time going in and out because of the anesthesia, the doctor entered with the results. At the time Tricia was out and he told me that it was cancerous, and I was now responsible for telling her the bad news upon her waking. Knowing that cancer was a possibility, still did not lessen the shock of her, my wife having cancer in her body. Before Dr. Gordon's departure, he informed me that all signs detectable of cancer was removed and that part of the lining of the stomach was also removed. My thoughts during Moments between Dr. Gordon speaking to me and Tricia waking was that she is in God's hand and that she will live through this. My faith had a battle with my fear. I had to pull on my faith, because this husband was in shock and multiple thoughts of fear were racing through my mind.

The time had come, Tricia was awakening and I knew she wanted to know. She opened her eyes and probably noticed the look on my face, so she asked the life changing question "What was it"? I told her it was cancerous and that he felt that he removed all that could be detected. It was amazing that she did not respond outwardly with any fear, just total strength. That Moment set the tone for the remainder of her treatment and recovery. Proud was not even close to what I felt towards her, it could not be put into words.

She proceeded to get physically stronger over the next few weeks leading up to the follow-up appointment with Dr. Gordon to discuss the next steps to take in the path to overcome this detour in her life. We met with Dr. Gordon and he gave her options to think about with chemo, even through this she saw her future life more than the current situation. I saw her kick in and say "there are challenges ahead and I will make it through." This was evident by two facts as with chemo treatment becoming a certainty. She first decided to delay the start of her first chemo treatment so she could attend a weeklong intensive class session in Lynchburg Va., for the Master's program in which she was enrolled through Liberty University. She was not going to allow her graduation plans to be delayed, she was going to live. The second astonishing thought was that our son Brenton was in his senior year in college and his graduation date was set and she planned her chemo around his graduation because she was determined she would be there for him.

Often times she has called me her rock, but what I saw through the chemo, the recovery and the continued quest to live life, she could be called a whole mountain range. Tricia was diagnosed with stage 3-C ovarian cancer but she was more concerned about her family more than what she was going through. She has been amazing through it all. I watched her struggle with energy, losing her appetite, trying to go when the body said rest and losing her hair, but through it all she took living life to the fullest to above imagination proportion. She carried a constant smile, not fake at all; she was always trying to give encouragement rather than receive it. Yes, there were some very tough days, but she lived for the good days. During chemo times she had intraperitoneal chemo for two days and she had to lie down to receive it. She refused to wear the normal opened back hospital gowns, instead she went shopping for different fashionable gowns she could wear along with matching socks and jewelry. She chose to get out of the house and participate in society when the body allowed her to, knowing that soon this all will be a memory and a testimony for later. She turned her lemons into lemonade by being available to others who were going through cancer as an encourager, a voice of reason and hope to all. When she was younger, she had the nickname "Sunshine" which fittingly represents her even more now because that's what she has brought to others through the past four plus years. Of course as her husband this has not been easy for me either and I thought I was a very strong person, but she has pushed me to be stronger than I could have ever dreamed I could be. She has taken the role of Ovarian Cancer Awareness Ambassador as a purpose and shared her story to speak life to all that will listen. Through the whole ordeal, Tricia not only talks the faith, she walks the faith as she lives in the faith!

Tracy Aparicio Fogg, II
(Oldest Son of Gailtricia Fogg)

When I was eight years old, on September 30, 1996, I was run over by a car and suffered a brain injury and was not expected to live. I had to go to Scottish Rite Children's hospital in Atlanta. I came home on **December 20, 1996.** Although I was still somewhat comatose, my mother told me that she rolled me in front of the Christmas tree and told me that I was her Christmas present and that I would be alright. She knew that God would restore my faculties. Because of this, she keeps the Christmas tree up all year.

After my Mom had her surgery on December 14, 2011 she stayed in the hospital for several days. She came home on **December 20, 2011.** I reminded my mother that we came home on the same date. I told her, "Mom, you are our Christmas present!" She had a long road ahead of her too, just like I did. She did not give up on me and we were not giving up on her. I had no fear while my Mom was going through ovarian cancer. While my Mom was in the state of recovering, she had angels watching over her, she's a strong woman spiritually and we wouldn't let her give up even if her body wanted her to. As long as she had Jesus on her side we all knew that she would be good to go. She would live! She was willing to let God work through her and that's the name of the game.

Brenton Fogg
(Youngest Son of Gailtricia Fogg)

As my mother went through ovarian cancer, it was very hard for me at first! I was thinking like, "How could my mama have cancer?" Once I looked at my daddy's face and tears began to roll down his eyes after telling me, I really felt that this was very serious and that I had to step up and really help! It was very hard to watch my mother go through everything from losing her hair to being very weak. But after watching how her attitude was about it, I felt better! She handled it like a champ and I knew that she wanted us to take it like a champ too, so I did! Instead of being sad about it, we used this situation to encourage others, everywhere we went! I knew that GOD was going to take care of all of us, so my worrying days were over!

Robin Tutt Mole
(Friend of Gailtricia Fogg)

Gailtricia journeyed through the healing of ovarian cancer with determination and unwavering faith. She exhibited a strong intimacy with God. Gailtricia listened untiringly to Christian tapes to continue to strengthen her faith. She prayed that God would continue to keep her mind in line with what the Bible said about healing. After surgery, she went to Virginia for class, exercising her strength which God has given her. She viewed everyday as a day closer to the last day of chemotherapy. Her theme of prayer was "no pain, no complications and no disease left in her body". She was transparent with her family and close friends and made sure they knew how her progress was going. Gailtricia physically loss weight, loss her hair and loss her appetite. However, she accessorized her beauty with her own style of hats matching with her outfits and jewelry. She made losing your hair just simply gorgeous! Gailtricia has taken this journey through ovarian cancer as a pathway to help and encourage others who are diagnosed with ovarian cancer. She has spoken to many community groups and has traveled to tell her story. Gailtricia has and continues to network with other ovarian cancer survivors. She has a strong desire to bring more awareness of ovarian cancer the city of Macon. She has taken this healing as a stepping stone used by God to help others.

Carol Spain
(Friend of Gailtricia Fogg)

My God-sister, Gailtricia Fogg was diagnosed with Ovarian Cancer December 14, 2011, eight months after my mother died. It was very hard for me because my mom, Ruby Spain was an Ovarian Cancer survivor of 20 years when she died April 15, 2011. Just like Tricia, my mom was a trooper. She had colon cancer and a year before she died the ovarian cancer returned.

Tricia, as we call her always kept the Faith. She was a joy through all of her trials. She always had a smile to give, as she does now, no natter what. I don't know anyone who is joyful all the time, other than Tricia. Tricia was a very caring person even through her sickness. During this time, Tricia's mother, Mattie Thomas was going through Dementia. She was still there to help her mother anyway she could, even though I know this had to be tough for her in her sickness as well, we never knew it. She is such an inspiration to all!

Chapter 16

God's Handiwork

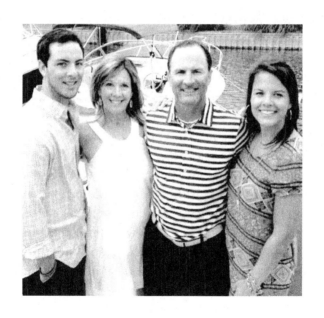

By Betsy Gentry

I have been an incredibly healthy person all my life - no issues other than the occasional cold, a few aches, and only in the hospital to have babies. My diet has almost always been healthy (although, I do love a good burger and fries!), I exercise frequently, I play golf and tennis, and there is very little stress in my life. I even took vitamins for women over 50! I was doing everything right as far as doctors and health magazines were concerned.

Then in April 2015 I began having some annoying stomach issues - some pain and bloating. Initially, I chalked it up to some medicine I was taking for carpal tunnel, but one night it got particularly bad. I was at my doctor's office first thing the next morning and she sent me off to the emergency room thinking it was appendicitis.

Here's where I began to take notice of all of God's handiwork in what was about to happen… My admitting nurse in the ER was a woman I've known for several years. She was so good about making sure we were taken care of and were getting all our questions answered. I had a CT scan so they could check my appendix. However, instead of getting wheeled into surgery, I was handed a phone where my Ob/GYN gave me the news that they had seen what looked like a tumor on one of my ovaries. Her words were, "We're concerned it might be ovarian cancer." My husband who was with me fell apart, but I'm pretty sure I was just in shock. I took down the names and phone numbers of the oncologist she wanted me to see, set up an MRI for later in the week, and then was sent home. In my mind, though, her words "might be" were a beacon of hope to me ---even though the world had started shattering around me--- it wasn't yet a sure thing.

That was the day I stepped off the cliff into the world of cancer. My family came with me. It's just a crazy thing - one minute your life is normal and your days are spent doing whatever little things seem to be important - and then, life as you know it ends and you begin doing whatever you need to do to make more of those days take place, and to fill them with what actually matters. And so it began.....

The next week was spent getting medical tests, seeing new doctors (I had never been to an oncologist before), and figuring out what came next. At my first visit to my oncologist, I walked into a waiting room with a number of women in various stages of either baldness, scarves, or wigs. I knew immediately that I didn't belong to their "club" and that this was all going to be all right. A tumor isn't always cancer - right?

I was scheduled for a complete hysterectomy in May. Prior to that, an MRI showed 2 more tumors - now I'm up to three, but praying that they could all be benign. I do believe in the power of prayer, and I had a whole lot of people asking God to take care of me! While they had me opened up to take out all my "lady parts" and appendix, they saw that my gall bladder was a disaster. Apparently it's supposed to look like a wet balloon and mine had so many stones it looked like a porcupine. In hindsight, it was probably my nasty, porcupine-like gall bladder that sent me to the emergency room initially, which means it saved my life! Ovarian cancer is a silent killer - usually no symptoms until it has spread. So I thank God for my nasty gall bladder (which had to be removed by a different surgeon).

My husband Jeff, told me the first thing I asked him when I woke up after surgery was, "Do I have cancer?" He thought that was a forgone conclusion, but I was very hopeful. Unfortunately, it was cancer, but the surgeon was able to remove all visible traces. They did find cancer cells in 2 of 20 lymph nodes, though. So, a week after surgery I met with the oncologist to discuss treatment.

Getting the pathology report (Ovarian Cancer Stage 3b) was like receiving the cancer diagnosis the first time. I naively hoped that the fact that they "got it all" meant that I was free of this disease.

Sadly, it seems I have an aggressive form, and because it was in lymph nodes chemo would be necessary. Looking back, I think I would have been worried not to have had any form of treatment because that's the only way I could FIGHT this nasty disease instead of just hoping it didn't attack again.

Time to side track to my family and my support system. I'm married with two adult children. My daughter was living at home at the time, and my son lived 4 hours away in Charlotte. I have never known the depth of love that I have for those three amazing people. I thought I loved them before, but once you see what you may lose - or better yet, how wonderful the people closest to you are - there is an incredible burst of love for them every day! We had so many more heart-felt conversations, hugged longer, listened carefully, and talked with each other more - it's like Tim McGraw's song "Live Like You Were Dying"… every moment with each person you love is even sweeter when you can't take it for granted!

My friends were also amazing! There were meals, cards, flowers, phone calls, texts, and most importantly, prayers. I now realize these are God's angels who walk us through what we could never get through on our own. For anyone who is facing cancer without faith in God, I don't know how you can do it. I was given just the right person, phone call, note, etc. at just the right times. My family experienced the same thing. God put people in their paths who genuinely had just the right thing to say, the right shoulder to lean on. Too many details to go into here, but trust me when I say that God's handiwork was absolutely amazing to experience!

So, after the surgery and diagnosis, the fight begins. Here's another part of stepping off the cancer cliff into a world you never thought you'd experience. There are different doctors, different terminology, different medications, different words and experiences that didn't exist before. Suddenly you have to become an expert on things you don't understand, but it's your fight and you have to arm yourself with everything you can. We spoke to a number of different doctors about treatment options - my vocabulary and science knowledge had to expand in a matter of a couple of weeks. My family's regular life turned into a world of science with me, and off we went....

My treatment plan was to have IV and IP chemo treatments of Taxol and Cisplatin. IV is traditional chemo done through a chest port leading to a vein. IP is a special kind of fun - it is given through a port in your belly that sends the toxic warriors (chemo) directly into the peritoneum. But first, I had to go to "cancer school" (my term) where I was given an incredible amount of information about what chemo can/will do, how treatments work, what to eat, what not to eat, what to do, what not to do, and what some (but not all) of the side effects could be. It was here that the nurse gave me an idea of when my hair would begin to fall out. Now, there was a day circled on my calendar! Suddenly that was all I could think about! Once the hair goes, everyone knows you have cancer, right?

I made an appointment with the "Woman's Place" in the hospital for a wig fitting. It's important to go when you still have hair to make sure you look as close to normal as possible. I took 4 of my good girlfriends and my daughter. The wig they chose for me was like my hair, but better! It looked like I had walked right out of the salon. I chose a synthetic wig because they don't need styling, and you only need to wash them once a month (after all, if you don't have hair to wash, you don't want to be styling someone else's hair - this is your hall pass for several months!). It was expensive and I'm still irritated that my insurance company didn't pay for it because they said it was cosmetic. But it was an important investment - I wore it pretty much every day for about 8 months. More on that later....

One of the first things I recommend to women (or anyone) diagnosed with cancer is to immediately find support and information. I asked my doctor to put me in touch with someone who had been through my exact treatment (she was a wonderful help and we are

147

still in touch). I got involved at the Cancer Support Center which has so much to offer for those recently diagnosed through long-term survivors. If you don't live in an area that has access to something similar, find an on-line group, or somewhere that you can talk, share information, get answers, etc.

Another thing that was so helpful for my family was the CaringBridge website. I have to admit that setting up a site like that with my name on it was very emotional --- I have followed a number of people on the site - some of whom are no longer with us. But, in our case, it was the best way to get information and updates out to people who cared about us. Prior to that, any time my husband, Jeff or the kids were out, they spent so much time giving people the same stories, updates, answering the same questions. This made it much easier on them! It was also helpful to me to be able to express what was really going on - the good and the not-so-good - and to continue to thank those who were walking through this with us. People can also add comments on the site, so reading those was one more measure of support that helped get me through.

Back to pre-treatment. Before the chemo can begin, the ports must be put in. I had heard this was a pretty simple, easy and painless event. Not so much in my case. They had to implant my two ports in two procedures. The anesthetic seemed to be just fine when they inserted the chest port. However, with my stomach port I could feel things AND hear the radiologist saying he couldn't find exactly where to put it. Kind of creepy, but eventually it was in, and I was out!

My first chemo treatment began 5 days after my ports were put in, but I've heard of several people who start it the day after getting their ports. They are better people than I! I needed a few days to catch my breath. I was very emotional the day of my first treatment - but I wasn't particularly anxious or nervous. God was again taking really good care of me - I was holding tightly on to His hand and following His lead. It took a couple of hours before I was actually getting chemo. The first step is the pharmacist spending a LOT of time talking about each drug, possible side effects, etc. Then there is the "pre-game cocktail" of steroids, anti-nausea, and (in my case) Ativan. I highly recommend the Ativan - especially for the first chemo session. I thought they would give me a pill before they poked me and sent the drugs in, but it is given as an IV with the rest of the pre-game goodies. But, I will tell you that you can feel it the second it kicks in and it feels like you've just had 2 glasses of wine — really relaxed, no anxiety (but also a little difficulty not slurring your words). I continued having the Ativan with each chemo treatment - it really made it easier for me (and I'm no martyr!). Just sayin'…. for me, it was the ticket!

So the crazy thing about the chemo drugs are that the nurses who administer them have to put on Haz-Mat suits and masks when they are giving them because of their toxicity. Yet, that's what's going into your body to "heal you". It's crazy. I did think of each of the chemo treatments as my warriors, though, going into battle against this awful disease. I was rooting for them at every treatment!

One very cool thing was that my kids sent out emails to my friends, family, and pretty much anyone I'd ever met, soliciting short videos for me to watch during each of my treatments. It almost made me look forward to my chemo treatments knowing I would have some great, fun, creative videos that people took time to make to cheer me up. My daughter parceled out about 3 new ones to me each session and it made it less horrible to be there. As it turned out, a couple of people knew celebrities, sport stars, or solicited someone in the public eye that they had record a video for me. That was really cool, too! "Operation Chemo Cheer" was just one more thing that bolstered me through - and I still love going through the videos today! If you are a caregiver, consider this - people were so responsive and it made a huge difference every time I showed up for my chemo.

My chemo cycle was 2 days/week, 1 day the following week, then a week off. Each session was about 5 hours and I was blessed to have chemo buddies who took me, stayed with me (even though I slept a good bit of the time), and chatted and distracted me. It meant the world to me that people would take a day out of their time to do it, but I realize people genuinely want to help, and that when you are at your lowest, you need to accept the help.

Typically I felt pretty good the first couple of days after treatment (the steroids help that), then lousy and tired about 3 days after. I had to get used to not being able to be as active as I had been - that was a big lesson for me to learn. I had to learn to listen to my body and stay put, stay in pj's, just sit or lie down, when things got to be too much. Friends had set up a meal schedule online and it was such a blessing not to have to grocery shop or cook - especially on the days that were really grueling. Some of the time I had no appetite but I knew my family was fed. That's one of the best things your friends can do is put together a schedule for meals, rides, help in any way. You need to be able to accept help...people WANT to help and during chemo it's so welcome!

Three things I did during chemo that I know helped me get through it without major issues:

1. Drink water constantly. Staying hydrated makes a big difference, and I believe it helps flush out the toxins following chemo.
2. Eat a healthy diet. I didn't have a huge appetite but I did love the comfort food. Unfortunately it created a big constipation issue that sent me to the ER after my first week of treatments. Details are not necessary, but make sure you are eating less cheese and pasta, and eat more green, leafy vegetables and fruits.
3. Walk every day. Keep moving your body even when it doesn't seem like you're doing much of anything. I tried to get on the elliptical for 20-30 minutes each day (no resistance) even on chemo days. Usually I would come home from chemo and nap

for an hour or two, but then I would walk. Again I think it helps release the toxins, and your body just needs to keep moving to recover from this treatment. You may not be able to do it every day, but try to make it a habit.

Back to hair loss. I was more anxious and nervous about losing my hair than almost anything else. But, the thought of losing it is so much worse than when it actually happens. I went to the place I got my wig and they buzzed my hair while I still had a good bit. You never know what shape your head is until you are bald (or very closely shorn). It's a weird feeling and look! That was the day I started wearing my wig. Like I said, my hair has never looked as good as my wig, so I was feeling pretty good about myself. The only thing with the synthetic wig is that you shouldn't open a hot oven or a hot dishwasher while you're wearing it, so my daughter put a note on our oven that said "Beware of Hair" as a reminder.

My hair did gradually begin to fall out about two weeks after the nurse had told me it would. My scalp was kind of tingly during this time. I never lost every single hair - I had a few sprouts and my son called me "Tweetie Bird". I never could get the hang of tying scarves, so when I wasn't wearing my wig (which I pretty much just did for "fancy" occasions), I wore what I called tube tops - just a tube-shape of material that stretched over the head and was tucked in at the bottom. I also wore a little stocking cap at night while my hair was coming out so I didn't find hair all over my pillowcase in the morning.

There are several good things about hair loss once it actually happens. Really! First of all, the eyebrows and eyelashes are the last to leave and the first to come back after chemo. So for the most part, you can rock the baldness - I had a few friends who never wore a wig, they just looked edgy and cool. But to get a little more personal - once your hair falls out (and I mean you are just like the day you were born.....everywhere!), your shower time is so short, getting ready time is minimal, and when you have to pack to go somewhere, you travel VERY light! One weird thing that no one tells you though - all your nose hairs fall out, which doesn't feel like a big deal until there is NOTHING to stop your nose from running and it just leaks!

Again, my words of wisdom to anyone facing this is this: the thought of losing your hair is infinitely worse than when it actually happens. Grieve it, then go on. You are fighting a BIG battle and that's a minor casualty. It will return, you will get through it. In the meantime, rock your bald head, your alter-ego wig, whatever makes you feel good about yourself.

That's another thing about chemo. Everyone is different. You will be told of all kinds of side-effects. It reminded me of being pregnant when I was told all the possible issues I could face. Everyone is different, everyone's experience is different. I was so blessed to have had a "good" experience with my chemo. There were a number of issues I had been warned of, and ready for, that didn't take place - thank you, God!

Back to the chemo thing. One of the other things my wonderful family did was to create the Chemo Tracker. We have a plate in our kitchen that is usually reserved for writing "Happy Birthday" or "Welcome Home"....it became the mathematical calculation that was displayed in our house and on CaringBridge on how far in to chemo we were. Another thing to look forward to with each chemo session was that the Chemo Tracker was going to be updated!

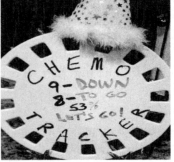

My chemo went on for a little over 5 months. The nurses who work in oncology are the best. I had some of the most caring people each time. Big shout out to those of you who work in this field. It must be tough and I know there are no holidays or weekends. Those of us who are on the receiving end appreciate everything you do to make the chemo experience a little better than it could be.

On my last day I was ready to ring the bell which I had seen from all the cancer patients I had followed. One problem was that my place didn't have a "bell". So I took my own "bedazzled school bell" that a friend had given to me. I slapped that thing over and over to celebrate in the infusion center. Little did I know that a friend and my daughter had me covered already. On the way home, my husband pulled the car into our church parking lot at which time the chapel bells started ringing! I was (and am whenever I remember it) a puddle of tears in thankfulness!

Eventually, and finally, chemo ended. It's as much a cause for celebration as it is scary. No longer are you fighting this disease. From this point, you just wait and pray that it doesn't come back. When I had my first scan following chemo it showed no evidence of cancer. That was the day I truly learned the meaning of "overjoyed". I had so much joy I couldn't contain it! I'm pretty sure that was the first time I exhaled in 8 months. I was an emotional basket case.

So that's the best - and the scariest - day since you stepped off the cancer cliff. Now you're cancer-free, but what do you do to stay there? Every day you hear things you should do, need to do, don't do, etc. Seems like everyone you talk to is an authority on what to do. I believe everyone needs to decide what will work best in their situation and do their best to remain healthy. At the same time, many of us were healthy going into this, so it's up to each individual to decide what will/should/can work for them.

I had genetic testing done after my diagnosis and the good news is that I don't have a gene I'm passing on to my children (or anything my family needs to be concerned about). The bad news is that

Ovarian cancer is only genetically carried in about 15% of cases. So, it's scary to think you could be doing everything "right" and this still happens.

My next steps are these: I will do whatever I can to help those who are diagnosed, give information to those with vague symptoms who don't know what to look for in this horrible silent disease, raise money for a test for this horrible disease, and work to stay healthy for a long, long time. Sadly, there is a high probability of recurrence for me, but I will continue to pray for complete and total healing for me and so many others.

To wrap up my story, I am BLESSED! Isn't that crazy? But I really see it! Before this horrible diagnosis, I didn't see all the things I do today. My family is closer than ever, my friends have seen the strength that I have drawn from them and my faith in God. I have a new outlook - and I know every day is a gift!

Chapter 17

My Intent for the
Remainder of My LIFE

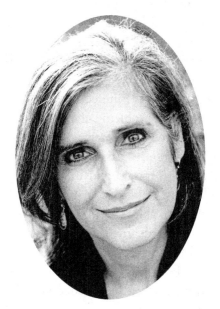

By
Halle Reid Holland
Rich Holland
Aleah Holland James

A summary of my perspective on my reoccurrence of Ovarian Cancer: The reality of the state of my body and my intent to create a more connected mind & spirit collaboration!

This piece is written to frame my intent for the remainder of my life. It does not suggest that these views are right for others. Everyone's situation is different, as is how they must handle it. This is simply my personal statement.

It is my lifelong observation -- not just now during cancer time -- that my body is very highly influenced by my state of my mind (perspectives and thoughts) and my spirit (including personality and natural inclinations). Recently, however, these dimensions appear unusually out-of-sync. While my mind and spirit are generally energetic, creatively minded, inquisitive, and attracted to the challenge and play of problem-solving, my body just seems to be less able to keep up (or is too easily sidelined by life, or perhaps the intensity of these interests, drives and even inherit unconscious motivations.) More simply said and in a perhaps silly metaphor: I feel now a bit like a three-legged young dog – a little bit cute but unable to fully run, skip and play to the degree I'd like to – and, incidentally, to the degree that I physically feel I'm meant to. But having said that, it is my clear intent to conduct my life with a leaning toward running, skipping, and playing as I can best manage it, making adjustments as needed, and for me that means full engagement with family, friends, meaningful work, church, adventuring a bit, and often learning/trying new things.

Therefore, all treatments and decisions about life management must carefully consider the needs of the three dimensions and integrate healthy choices to each, and with an eye for a collective balance and synergistic effect on all. My goal is to lead a healthy and productive life, and through my actions, influence the same for my family.

To be clear, my philosophy about the future and my cancer plan is really not about "getting as many years as I can." To me, that is silly. However, I am seeking to continue to grow as a person and to contribute as much as I can to the people I love in spite of the backdrop of this disease. I seek to create quality experiences in this life, to the best of my abilities, for as long as that is possible. So, I am seeking to surround myself with a constellation of people and resources who will help me:

- Be informed, analytical, forward-looking and creative about treatment options and life-style changes; Factor in and grow in the immense realm of spirituality and all it means;

- Stay calm for myself and radiate calm to others to ensure that my family, friends and colleagues' experience of my cancer leans more to the peaceful side than the agitated or sad one;

- Resist assumptions about how this illness stereotypically defines my ability or willingness to live well; and

- Find courage when I need it at the most tender Moments, receive straight-talk when I need to hear it, and be open to inspiration, often found in the tiniest of places or ways.

The miracle I'm seeking is not necessarily to live an astonishing long life against the odds, but rather to live the years I have in a quality, loving, peaceful, productive, and fun way.

Rich Holland
(Husband of Halle Reid Holland)
Fall, 1973 - Discovering Halle Reid

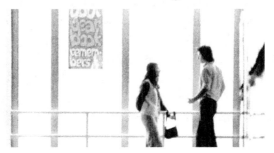

When I was 15, I dated a girl with quite a dramatic personality. Before Christmas, I searched for the right present for her and ended up buying what I thought was a striking, ornately-designed top. I was sure she would like it. She didn't. Truthfully, the gift was cheap - I got it at one of those mall bazaar carts, but I learned a valuable lesson that Christmas – the most special people in your life love you for who you are and not for what you can give them.

I found that special a girl at our high school Drama Club's performance of "The Children's Hour." Halle Reid was captivating; a sophomore beauty with long brunette hair who seemed to delight in the role she was playing. She was "alive" on stage and I was very intrigued. Aside from this dramatic role, Halle went on to be our Chorus President, school TV news anchor, and representative to Presidential Classroom. She was smart, kind, confident, humble, and had strong values. She was pretty too, and it didn't take long to fall in love with her. After dating for just one year, I knew I wanted to marry her. At 17, beginning college in the fall, marriage remained a distant, but patient thought in the back of my mind for the next five years.

After I graduated from Miami University, I proposed to Halle in the summer before her senior year at M.U. I had no money, wouldn't begin teaching until the Fall, and didn't have a clue about buying an engagement ring. Instead, we bought a couch! She said yes to my proposal and while I know she would have liked an engagement ring, she never said a word about it. This was a girl who loved me for who I was and not for the things I could give her. We married on May 16, 1980.

I share this part of our story because it is as important as our chapter with cancer. Those precious Moments are indelibly etched in my memory. We loved each other for a very long time and I will eternally love her. By the way, Halle finally got a diamond engagement ring, though she never asked for it and loved me as if she didn't need it.

Funny Girl

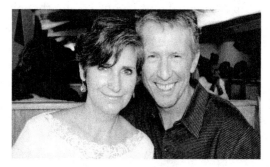

We of course had tough and trying Moments – Moments that brought tears and sobriety, but we also shared Moments in which humor and laughter helped us withstand the trials. She was brave – and funny!

After her initial surgery, during the resulting 10-day hospital stay, the Hospital Pastoral Counselor came to see her. His charming bedside manner began with, "Now, you have to learn to say those three words!" (I have cancer) He obviously was someone who relished his role helping cancer patients figure out the God-awful obvious truth of their condition. Not impressed with his inane prompt, knowing what he expected her to say, Halle responded,

"I am hungry?" I'm sure the brilliant counselor was stupefied by her response. This was so typical of Halle – simple, grounded, practical, and funny!

Years later after experiencing some discomfort in her stomach, we went to the emergency room. While waiting for the results of her blood test, we were getting hungry so Halle suggested that my son and I go to Wendy's and get something to eat, and bring a cheeseburger back for her. We did and she enjoyed her cheeseburger in the triage room. When the doctor came in (with the test results showing a gall bladder gone bad), he looked at the Wendy's wrapper and then at her as she finished the last bite and said, "You did not just eat that!" to which Halle replied, "I did and it was delicious!" The doctor was mad as a hornet, but after he left the three of us just laughed and laughed. She thought that irony was so funny. She was irrepressible! Brave and funny! She was wonderful!

Aleah Holland James
(Daughter of Halle Reid Holland)
Considerations for BRCA1

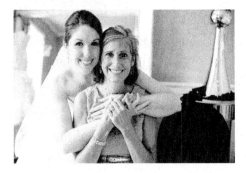

My Mom, Halle Reid Holland, was diagnosed with ovarian cancer at the age of 51 in December 2008. She went to heaven in August 2013. Throughout her battle with cancer, she endured chemos, radiation, multiple surgeries (including a craniotomy), easily 50-60 lung drains, an oxygen tank, an incorrect diagnosis which removed her gall bladder, and the loss of all of her hair. Throughout all of the pain and indecencies, she managed her situation and those around her with incredible grace and profound humor. She was determined to live whatever time she had on earth as a complete person that would continue to grow and contribute to the world around her. She sought quality of life, understanding very realistically that quantity of life may not be her option.

On July 16, 2009 Mom got the report back that she had the BRCA1 gene mutation, which predisposes one for ovarian and breast cancers. I can imagine her referring to this gene as "wonky," a testament to her always perfectly timed wit and unique interpretation of life. This gene, coupled with years of stress and other factors, was likely part of the causation for her cancer.

- 12% of women will develop breast cancer in their lifetime. 50-65% of those diagnosed with the BRCA1 genes will develop breast cancer by age 70. It is slightly less for BRCA2.

- 1.3% of the general population will develop ovarian cancer in their lifetime. 39% of those with BRCA1 will develop ovarian cancer by age 70.[1]

Mom immediately began reaching out to all of our female relatives to make them aware that BRCA1 was present in our family line. These conversations revealed great aunts and grandmothers that had died from breast or undiagnosed ovarian cancer. As we began to piece together the potential significance of this gene in our family tree, she reassured me that I did not need to find out then if I had it. I did a CA-125 blood test to evaluate the cancer antigen 125 in my blood to tide us over. It came back at a "5," so we moved on with a sigh of relief.

In summer 2015, I was on the way to a wedding reception when my aunt (my Mom's younger sister) called me to let me know that

[1] "BRCA1 and BRCA2: Cancer Risk and Genetic Testing." *National Cancer Institute*. National Cancer Institute. April 1, 2015. Web. June 29, 2015.

she had pursued genetic testing, and it came back positive for the BRCA1 gene mutation. She was moving forward with genetic counseling to decide where to go from there, now needing to evaluate if she should need to go as far as a double mastectomy a la Angelina Jolie.

The next day, I began to consider whether or not I should get the test done myself. If both my Mom and aunt have it, my risk is likely greater. Genetic counseling and testing as it relates to BRCA appeared to be (at a quick glance) covered by my insurance. The relatively new Genetic Information Nondiscrimination Act (GINA) had made it illegal to be "discriminated" against by employers and health insurance providers due to a genetic condition, which included denial of coverage or the raising of rates. The opportunity to prepare my mind and begin to systematically evaluate my health as it related to breast and ovarian cancers seemed like the reasonable and logical path to pursue.

Despite the logic, I was afraid. I did not want to rush my husband and my desire for kids, nor rush into surgeries I may not even truly need. I didn't (and still don't) want to live in fear, but also did not want to be ignorant or blind to what very well could be my reality too. I was already vigilant, but also scared. With there being no currently effective prescreening methods for ovarian cancer (only wildly subtle symptoms), the non-surgical options currently available for me to monitor for and address the disease have no effect on decreasing the mortality rate. I knew that the test coming back positive for the mutation did not guarantee that I would develop either cancer, but then again it would not be just "cancer" anymore: it would be a "genetic cancer syndrome" for me, and possibly for my kids.

Kids. My husband and I were not ready. I had always longed for kids and now I began to second-guess myself there too. Would it be fair of me to bring kids into the world and not know if I would be passing down a genetic predisposition for cancer? Would it be fair for me to bring kids into the world with the chance their Mom may not live 80+ years as hoped?

It was a lot of unknowns and a lot of what ifs. I suppose that is, in and of itself, typical of cancer: unknowns and what ifs. I decided, after seeking counsel from my closest friends and other family members that I would get the test done. At least if I knew, I would have all of the information and could make the most informed decision possible.

This, ladies and gentlemen, is why every health-related commercial on TV advises you to consult with your doctor or, in my case, nurse practitioner. I went into my next "lady doctor" visit prepared to have the genetic testing done. I voiced this to my wonderful NP, sitting very straight and trying my best to be brave. She listened carefully and supportively. Then she asked me: "What would you do right now if the tests came back positive?"

I thought about it. "I guess I don't know."

"Do you want kids?"

"Someday. Not right now."

"All right. Let's think this through."

She went on to tell me that my options in terms of preventative measures, at this time, would be surgery. Surgery would impede my ability to have kids. She also told me that though the GINA prevented employers from denying me health insurance or employment, having this test done could cost me something else very significant; life insurance. If I had this test done and came back positive (at age 28!), I could be deemed "too risky" an investment and denied life insurance for the rest of my life.[2]

[2] "If You Want Life Insurance, Think Twice Before Getting A Genetic Test." *Fast Company*. February 17, 2016. Web. August 24, 2016. http://www.fastcompany.com/3055710/if-you-want-life-insurance-think-twice-before-getting-genetic-testing..

163

This was, of course, the worst case scenario. But goodness, what a significant scenario. I immediately thought of my husband (and those future potential children) and feared for them if something ever happened to me. Here I was considering the likelihood something would happen to me, and it turned out that if I have this test done in advance, my family may not be taken care of when I'm gone because of a decision I'd made.

My Mom always had the keenest of forethought. She was so responsible that she planned out her entire memorial service in advance so that we would not have to worry about it amidst dealing with losing her. She was so "big picture" with her thinking that she planned to pay off my brother and my college debt with her life insurance, and then allocate an additional portion of that life insurance to be a "nest egg" for us as well. She intentionally worked to spare us from what all she was really going through, and she never complained. She made her decisions wisely, carefully. She made her decisions out of love and thoughtfulness for us, and it was important to me that I follow her example to demonstrate that well researched, well planned consideration for my family too.

I did not get the test that day. Once I've had my kids, my NP and I agreed we would revisit this conversation and move forward as necessary. I am grateful to my wonderful NP for not chastising me or pushing me in a way she thought I should go. Instead, she took the time to listen, ask questions, and discuss my options with me in a way that made sense to and for me. She assured me that we have time, a concept often foreign when cancer is involved.

I am even more thankful for my (wise, witty, devoted, kind, beautiful…) mother who made such a profound and lasting impact on me. Though her time on earth was shorter than most, she did a great deal with the time she had. Her love was boundless and is still felt by all who knew her. Cancer and the BRCA gene may have significantly impacted her life (and ours by association), but it never once defined her.

I will not let it define me either. All that I am and all that I have yet to do is so very much more than one "wonky" gene.

Chapter 18

Prayer Availeth Much

By Kelly Jackson

I am 40 years old, happily married for 10 years to my husband Mike, and mother to two beautiful daughters, Ella Murphy, age 9, and Hannah Rose, age 5. Mike and I had been married for 3 months when I began experiencing unusually harsh abdominal distress.

After consulting with our parents, Mike and I visited a physician. I underwent a series of physical exams, x-rays, CT scans, and other procedures. One doctor offered an opinion that I might have ovarian cancer. Needless to say, this opinion generated a great deal of concern amongst our families. An ensuing appointment with my OB/GYN resulted in discovery of a large mass in my right abdominal area that indeed "...might be ovarian cancer." We were referred to Dr. Jeffery Hines, a Gynecologic Oncologist. He described two masses to us and advised that they be removed as quickly as possible. He then asked the group to join him in prayer. The procedure was scheduled for April 21, 2006.

The surgery involved removing the 2 tumors. One of them was identified as being aggressively malignant. I was release from the hospital 8 days later. Due to the location of the tumors, we did not know if we would be able to have children. Dr. Hines encouraged us to try and, as I mentioned before, we have been blessed with two healthy daughters.

I have been cancer-free for 10 years and I am immensely grateful to God and to the skills and faith of Dr. Hines.

Chapter 19

Self-Diagnosing

By Allison Johnson

I went to my primary care doctor on a Tuesday afternoon in November, 2011, because what had been generalized discomfort for a while had become significant pain. For years, I had suffered from irregularity; for months I had a fullness in my abdomen that intermittently caught my attention; for weeks, I felt that my bowels were not fully evacuated; and for days, I'd actually experienced pain.

In fact, on the previous Sunday I was overcome with exhaustion and such generalized, severe pain causing me to be significantly frightened.

So, I thought ...
Diverticulitis?
Ovarian cyst?
Bladder cancer?
Mesothelioma?
(I had read So Much for That only a few months earlier.)

I went through all the options I thought fit my symptoms, then settled on diverticulitis.

I saw the PT in my doctor's office ... a wonderful young woman who had treated me for a number of minor illnesses over the past four or five years. When I told her about my symptoms, she immediately said, "I'm not sure what's going on, but you're not one to complain, so I'd like to get a CT scan."

The scan was scheduled for the next afternoon, and I went blithely back to my everyday obligations. But in the interlude between my appointment and my CT, I did further research, and decided that I had a prolapsed bowel, or one of the many related complications that seem to cluster in constipated women who have had hysterectomies.

In fact, in the hours after my scan was completed, I became convinced that I was suffering from a prolapsed bowel because of other symptoms

170

that I remembered, especially the generalized pressure on my entire pelvic floor whenever I tried to have a bowel movement.

Figuring that I'd likely be in for some sort of surgical intervention, but not dwelling on it, I moved forward into Thursday morning. At around 9 a.m. on Thursday, I received a call from the PT at my doctor's office, and she was just as breezy as could be ... an affect I now realize was a real effort. She first went through all that was unremarkable about my CT scan, which was quite a list. Then she rather casually mentioned that "the only remarkable findings on the scan were [and I could tell she was reading from the report] 'poorly circumscribed omental implants and a thickening in the peritoneum.'"

So do you know what the omentum is? I didn't. And although I knew what the peritoneum is, I didn't know what might cause "thickening."

As a result of my ignorance, when Lori (the PT) told me she and the doctor had consulted and wanted me to try to get in to see my gynecologist that same day, I was relatively nonplussed. AND I was confused. Once I looked up omentum, though, I began to understand that the possibilities were pretty serious. But since my college major was English, I decided to defer to the medical professionals ... at least for that day.

True to her word, Lori had reached someone in my gynecologist's office immediately. She faxed over all the reports, then called me back and told me that my gynecology group would be calling to set up an appointment. Within 30 minutes, the office called.

In the meantime, because the discomfort in my lower left abdomen and the urgent but ultimately misleading sense that I needed to void my bowels was fairly intense, I packed my computer and some projects that required my attention, and left my office for the day. Just as I was pulling out of the parking lot of the office, my phone rang. And that's when the stakes were raised.

171

A very sweet and pleasant woman, the nurse from my gynecologist's office candidly told me that they would gladly see me that day, but that they were going to want me to see a gynecologic oncologist as soon as possible, and inquired as to whether or not I could rearrange my schedule to go to Atlanta or Lawrenceville or Gainesville that afternoon.

Whoa.

I communicated relatively coherently with her, and continued to drive with some degree of caution (actually, I might have been reckless; I don't really know). But as the words of the nurse began truly to sink in, I became pretty frantic. When I remembered her offering to call in to the pharmacy something for the pain, it dawned clearly on me that we were not playing.

My best friend knew I was waiting for a call from our gynecologist's office, so she wasn't surprised when I called her to fill her in. She was floored, though, when I told her that since the last time we spoke, I had felt the focus of this whole process shift toward ovarian cancer. I didn't tell her that I was pretty sure it was Stage 3; that would really be stretching my medical credentials.

And I knew I could be wrong. But it was clear to me that there was something very serious going on, and that the two "remarkable" indications on the CT scan were related. It sure sounded like metastasis of some kind.

So as I was filling her in, I was overcome by the reality that I was driving toward home with a bomb that was going to rock my husband's world. He had already lost one wife to cancer; how could I tell him that another wife might be at risk? But how could I NOT tell him? And so I arrived home, filled him in, watched him purse his stiff upper lip, and when he asked me what I was going to do next, I replied, "I'm going to decorate the Christmas tree."

Of course, while I was looking at thirty years' accumulation of ornaments, I kept debating what I should do about contacting my daughter and son. I have an understanding with both that I won't keep things from them, and that I'll trust them to handle any bad news that concerns them. But what could I tell them? There was nothing definitive at that point, and they were in Vermont and California. What good would it do for them to worry with no focus for their concern?

I settled this dilemma by telling myself I would call them as soon as I consulted the oncologist, which the nurse had indicated she hoped could be scheduled either that day or the next. About the time I reached some peace about the decision, the phone rang again. It was my gynecologist's office, with the disheartening news that, because of the backlog of post-Thanksgiving appointments, I couldn't be seen by an oncologist until Tuesday. I asked her if she thought I should try to get in to see another group, and she replied that perhaps my PCP could pull some strings to get me scheduled somewhere, but that, in the meantime, she would send my records over to the office at which she had made my Tuesday appointment.

The weekend that followed was, of course, the longest weekend of my life. I grew more bloated by the hour, and by Saturday night, looked like I was in the third trimester of a pregnancy. I now understand that the ascites were accumulating at a very rapid rate, and that my condition was approaching a very serious point.

When I went in to see the gynecologic oncologist on the following Tuesday, he conducted a thorough and pretty uncomfortable exam, and confirmed that he could feel a number of nodules that corresponded with images from the CT scan. And although he said he wouldn't call the nodules "cancer" until after he had a pathology report, he said that the nodules likely originated in the ovary, residual Fallopian tube, or the peritoneum. In retrospect, I know that he knew I had ovarian cancer; the only question left for him to answer for himself at that point was the typology and staging.

Although things were moving way too fast for my emotions to keep up, I know I was lucky to be scheduled for surgery so expeditiously. From the time my CT report was shared with me until the day of surgery, I had to wait only a week. My symptoms were worsening, and I'm not sure I could have waited much longer.

Although the procedure took longer than anticipated, it was apparently a major success. The surgeon deemed my debulking surgery "optimal," saying that he was able to remove all the lesions that were spread throughout my abdominal organs, with the exception of one small patch on my colon and he was confident that chemotherapy would take care of that remaining lesion.

The eight days I spent in the hospital are mostly a blur. I know that my husband and children took turns sitting with me, and that at no point did they leave me completely alone. I remember walking the halls with my IV pole, determined to get my strength back as quickly and completely as possible. I remember being absolutely stunned that my life had taken this dramatic and completely unanticipated turn.

In the weeks and months that followed, I would realize that I actually experienced traumatic shock when I received my diagnosis, and that the draconian nature of the debulking surgery only added to the trauma. It seems no exaggeration at all to me to say that a devastating diagnosis like cancer can lead to post-traumatic stress symptoms; I lived through such symptoms.

However, I ultimately overcame the post-traumatic shock and the depression and the despondency. I remember saying to my family pastor (and to anyone else who was within an earshot), "I just don't believe this is going to end badly any time soon. I just don't believe God is done with me yet."

These were unexpected words for me. I was not in the practice of framing my life in faith-based language; I wasn't even sure what I believed. But in the Moment of my greatest existential fear, I knew for certain that I had, to paraphrase Robert Frost, miles to go before I slept.

And that belief has been validated over and over again in years since my initial diagnosis. As I compose this account, I am four years and seven months A.C. (After Cancer). I had a seventeen-month remission after frontline treatment, and since completing treatment for a recurrence in 2013, have enjoyed dancing with N.E.D. (No Evidence of Disease) for twenty-eight months.

Time will tell whether I'm cured. I know without doubt that I am healed.

I am living more fully and joyfully than ever before. I don't know what the future holds, but today is beautiful.

Chapter 20

In the Best Shape of my LIFE

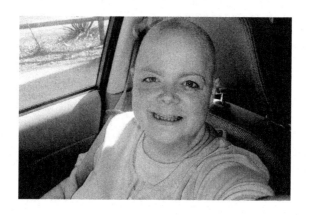

By Michelle Lawrence

At 42 years old I was in the best shape of my life, having lost 107 pounds and a very active yoga practice. It was early December, when my husband and I decided to get our Christmas gear out of the shed, and do some organizing. Towards the end of the afternoon, I had some stomach pain. I didn't think much about it, because I'd been working hard and lifting some heavy things. It wasn't even pain really, but more of a pulling sensation. A few days went by and the pulling sensation didn't ease up. I thought that I had pulled the mesh from an earlier hernia repair, so I made an appointment to see my doctor. I was sure they were going to tell me that that indeed was the problem. My doctor, actually, a PA/physician's assistant, listened to me and set up a CT scan. I don't know why, but an intense anxiety was taking over. I had nightmares before the appointment, and serious butterflies in my belly the morning of the scan.

The results came back quickly, an 8cm cyst on my left fallopian tube. My PA wasted no time in making me an appointment with the local OB/GYN. In fact, she made it for the very same day of the call. The OB/GYN did an internal exam and told me that my uterus was swollen, very swollen. He said it was the size of someone who was four months pregnant, and that I was in need of a hysterectomy. I had no idea what to make of that information. He set me up for some blood work and an ultra sound for the following day. Proceeding that visit, was an appointment to go over the results and fill out pre-op paperwork. I won't lie, I was nervous. I was not surprised that I needed a hysterectomy as I had had trouble with massive clots, and extended periods for a long time. My Mom went to the appointment with me. I remember sitting on the exam table in one of those lovely gowns that they give you and my Mom asked why I was so nervous. I told her that I was so afraid that he would tell me I was full of cancer. She said, "Did he give you any reason to think it would be cancer?" I took a deep breath and said, "No." About a minute later the nurse came in the room and told me to get dressed and go across the hall to the doctor's office. My first thought was that he was going to tell me that he couldn't do the surgery because I was too fat. Even though I had lost over 100 pounds, I still was not at my goal weight.

I walked into his office with my Mom right behind me. It was all paneled and filled with very large, dark bookcases. It was just beginning to get dark outside. I was seated across from my doctor with a large desk between us. He had his head down, looking at his hands. My Mom stood behind me with her hand on my shoulder. In a very soft voice, he said, "Can't do your surgery." I asked why, and he said that he ran a test called a CA-125 (Cancer Antigen 125), and that my numbers had come back abnormally high. I asked for more information, and was told that a normal number is 35 or less, mine had come back at over 500. He said he'd only ever seen that number higher once, over ten years ago. I still didn't get it. What was he telling me? I asked him what that meant. Very softly, head down again, he said, "I think you have ovarian cancer."

I remember that Moment so clearly, he wouldn't look at me. My Mom's hand tightened on my shoulder, and when I turned to look at her, there were tears streaming down her face. It was drizzling outside, the sky now black and the rain sparkling in the street lights. I felt ice in my body. Everything stopped. I remember thinking to myself.....ovarian cancer....isn't that the one they call the silent killer? The doctor pushed some papers towards me, a referral to a gynecological oncologist an hour and a half away from where I lived. There was a photo on one of the papers, but it was all mottled like a bad mimeograph. I could make out a male figure with a bow tie but that was it. My Mom continued to cry, and I remember telling her that we needed to think positive. I stood up, not really feeling my body, and said to the doctor, "I am fine right now, but in a few minutes, I'm not going to be. Can you give me something for that?" He wrote out a prescription and off we went into the night to get some Xanax.

Since my Mom had driven, I went back to her house where we sat at the dining room table and just looked at each other in silence. She called our priest and asked him to come over right away. I called my husband who was at work 2 hours away and when I heard his voice, I fell apart. Through sobs, I told him what had happened. He said he would be home as soon as he could and was leaving immediately. In the meantime, my priest came. He sat beside me at the table, and I'm sure he talked and prayed for me, but I can't tell you what he said as I didn't hear a word he said. He sat and looked at me as though he was expecting a response, but I had nothing to say. I apologized and he left. I took a Xanax and threw myself onto the couch facing the back, hiding my face from the world wishing for it all to go away. The next thing I know, Pete was there and he drove me home as I was in no shape to drive or be alone.

I don't remember the ride home or what we talked about when we got home. I do, however, remember that I cried all night. Pete would wrap his arms around me and all I could do was shake. It was the longest night of my life. Fear, and anxiety of the unknown was creeping in. Beast in the night.

An appointment was made for me to visit a gynecological oncologist 90 miles from our home. It was made for a few days later, and happened to fall on my husband's birthday. My Mom drove all three of us to the appointment. It is about a 2 hour drive, and I didn't say a word or open my eyes for the entire trip. I was deep in prayer. At the actual appointment, the oncologist was short with me. He asked why I was there, and why in the world would my local OB/GYN have sent me to him. I, of course, had no answer other than the report about the CA-125. The OB/GYN ONC scoffed and said that those numbers were useless, especially for a premenopausal woman such as myself. I didn't know what to say. He did an internal exam and since this was a teaching hospital, there were about 4 other strangers there watching. There I was in the stirrups and 5 strangers looking at my private parts. Just lovely. Later I would learn that you can request no students and no audience! Afterwards, the oncologist looked at me, and said he saw absolutely no reason to think that I had cancer. I asked if he would do the hysterectomy and he said he would.

Afterwards Mom, Pete and I went to Denny's. They were rejoicing. I was in disbelief. I kept asking, did he say, "No cancer?" This was to continue for another 3 weeks until the date of my surgery. It just didn't sink in. Later I had questions. What about my overly swollen uterus? No mention was made of that. As it turns out, the report about my uterus had not gotten to the oncologist before my appointment. I know this only because I got a letter about when to come into the hospital for my pre-op appointments for x-rays, an EKG, bloodwork and a biopsy of my uterus. Wait. What? They had received the information about my uterus and now wanted to check and see if there was cancer there. [Sigh] I was scared shitless.

On the day of the pre-op appointments, my Mom went with me. The biopsy was scheduled last. I asked my Mom to go with me to hold my hand. I was in tears before the doctor came in, but when she came in she was kind and compassionate. She hugged me and asked why I was scared and then showed me the equipment and told me what she was going to do, and how long it was going to take. I'll spare you the details but it wasn't pleasant in the least. Mom stood facing me, holding my hand and talked me through. Later she remarked about how she was surprised that I hadn't crushed the bones in her hand.

Now, came the waiting period for the results. My doctor had said he would call on Friday and he did. The conversation went exactly like this:

"May I speak to Michelle Lawrence please?"

"This is Michelle Lawrence."

"Hi Michelle. This is Dr. N. How are you today?"

"Nervous."

"Well, my news isn't going to help. You have uterine cancer. It's a ho-hum cancer, if you have any questions, call my nurse."

Click.

I did call the nurse who I have come to love over the years but on that day, she didn't have the answers I was looking for, only that it was a slow growing cancer. I had close to 3 weeks of time to wait until my surgery.

I think the waiting and not knowing was the absolute worst thing for me throughout this entire adventure. It still tortures my mind and creates an unimaginable amount of anxiety. My husband and Mom tried to get me to eat, but I just couldn't. They brought my favorite foods, and went out of their way to make some extra special homemade favorites, but I couldn't do it. I just couldn't. I lost 16 pounds in two weeks. Lack of food and nervous energy will do that to a body, and while I am always happy when I am able to lose some weight, this is not the way I would recommend doing it. The thing that finally got my body to accept food was the doctor telling me that I wouldn't be strong enough for surgery if I wasn't eating. It was still hard for me to deal with solid foods, so I was living on Ensure via a straw because...well, I wanted to have my surgery, and not complicate my chance of recovery.

This was also a time for both my husband I to say goodbye to our dream of having child. We had tried for years to have one on our own and finally had made peace with adopting a child. I didn't think anyone would let us adopt after receiving a cancer diagnosis. In the end, I had a complete hysterectomy and an abdominal wash. It took 6 tries to get the IV in and a call to the special IV team. I remember being wheeled into the operating room and being a sponge to hold on to. I felt myself drop it and tried to tell them but I was out. I woke up in the recovery room feeling like someone had kicked me super hard in the stomach but the nurses gave me pain meds that kicked in immediately. Not long afterwards my surgeon came in to see me. I'll never forget it. He said he had good news and bad news. The bad news is that I had uterine and ovarian cancer, spots found on both ovaries as well as in my uterus. The good news is that he was very confident that they got it ALL! He was jumping around like a little boy at a baseball game. I'll never forget it!

Turns out I am quite the happy soul on pain medication. The nurses kept me in ice chips and I was good. I was in recovery for 8+ hours because the hospital didn't have a bed for me. Eventually, they brought my mom and husband up to see me. It happened to be my nurse's birthday so I decided that was a great time for mom and I to sing Happy Birthday in our family tradition which means we sang in German! By the time I got a room, my husband had driven the two hours home to tend to the livestock and my mom had gone to her hotel room. The night was long but I was not in pain, just awake. The next morning a team of interns were making their rounds. They wouldn't tell me anything and when I asked if I was going to be ok they kept telling me to enjoy this day. I was terrified and in a fog from all the meds. I couldn't think clearly and wasn't remembering what my surgeon had said.

My surgery was on a Friday and I got to go home on Sunday afternoon. I have never in my life been so happy to be in my own space I met with my surgeon to learn the staging of my cancer. He said I has Uterine Cancer, Stage 1C and Ovarian Cancer, Stage 2B. The cancers were completely separate, there was no spread from one to the other. It is my understanding that this is quite rare. In fact, he told me that the uterine cancer saved my life as he was able to see/biopsy my ovaries when he removed my uterus. He removed all the staples and he told me 3 things were going to happen.

1. I was going to have chemotherapy.
2. I was going to have a port.
3. I was going to lose my hair.

I had the first chemo treatment via IV. I felt ok the first day but by day 3, I was unable to walk. It felt like someone was inside my leg bones with a baseball bat, trying to beat his way out. I had 3 really painful days with each treatment and by the time the 7th day came around I was feeling better. This happened for each of my 6 treatments.

My port was put in on March 1st, 2010. Everyone said it was nothing. I have one word for all those people. LIARS! I was not knocked out for this procedure but was taped to the table....a big X across my chest and my head taped so it was turned to the side. I remember all of it. Twilight drugs apparently don't work for me. I hated this procedure so much that now, 6 years later, I still have the port in my chest. I do what I need to do to maintain it and as long as it works, it will stay there. I NEVER want to have to have another port put in my chest as long as I live! I will say that I am SO glad I have my port, it made my chemotherapy treatments SO much easier and it kept my veins healthy as well.

On the day of my last treatment, my mom and I had made our usual trek. We'd drive down to the hospital and stay overnight at The House of Care. We had to be up early to be the clinic to have labs drawn before they would begin my 6 -8 hour infusion. Afterwards, because of all the steroids I had to take before chemo, I still felt grate and we' go out to dinner, stay over night one more night and then shop our way home for groceries and such. However, on the day of my last treatment, which was a Monday, my platelets had fallen to dangerously low levels and they refused to do the treatment. They told me to go home. I begged them to do it and get it over with. My hematologist said, "Honey, I'm trying to cure you, not kill you. GO HOME." So, we went home. No shopping this time, just me cursing up a blue streak. I was angry that I couldn't have my treatment and we'd have to go back AGAIN.

So, there I was, home on Tuesday morning when we should have been shopping our way home when the phone rang. It was our adoption agent. She said, "I have a 3 month old baby boy for you. Are you ready?" Without hesitation, I said, "YES!!!"

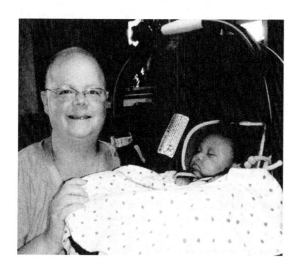

If my treatment had gone as planned, I would have been busy shopping and would have missed that phone call. Because this baby was an emergency placement, my agent would have had to have called the next family on the list. I firmly believe with all my heart that this was all in God's timing and He was telling me that it was time to close the door on cancer and take care of this sweet little baby. Four days later, we would take our son, Jeremiah Thomas Lawrence along with me for my last treatment. Because he was so young, I was not allowed to take him back into the treatment room with me but there were a string of nurses who came to the waiting room to great the newest member of our family.

It is now 6.5 years later and Jeremiah is in first grade. He sometimes comes to the clinic with me when I get my port flushed and to this day, the nurses all ask about him or come out to see him. In that time, I am beyond thankful to report that all my tests have come back showing that the cancer is gone.

I will forever be grateful for every single day I get to open my eyes. Every single night I stop by Jeremiah's bedroom to give him one last tuck in, a kiss and say a prayer of thanks for the blessing that is my son.

Chapter 21

Hope is Passion for What is Possible
"Live, Laugh and Love"

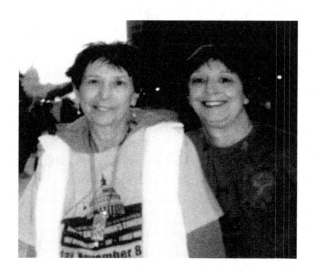

By Denise Lobodinski
(Sister of Reneé Lobodinski Specht)

When you first hear that a loved one has ovarian cancer, that is when your life will change forever in ways that you can never imagine. In January of 2005, my sister Reneé told me that she was tired and thought she had the flu. My response to Reneé was that she always got a yearly flu shot. I did not think about telling her to go to the doctor. Reneé like many women dealt with many issues with her husband and two children and was not as diligent about her own health.

In April 2005 she became very bloated and looked like she was pregnant. When she went to her internist the first thing they told her was that she had a bladder infection. Then she was sent to her gynecologist, who realized she had ovarian cancer. Her gynecologist did a PAP and it was completely normal and I keep telling women that ovarian cancer is not detected by a PAP test. Reneé was then sent to the Gynecological Oncology practice at Oklahoma University Medical Center. She was very fortunate that OU Medical was only ten miles from her home in Edmond, Oklahoma and had one of the best Gynecological Oncology groups in the country.

April 15, 2005 Reneé had a six hour surgery and during the surgery the surgeon discovered that the cancer had spread to certain organs in her abdominal area and she was diagnosed as having Stage 3C Ovarian Cancer. Unfortunately, she had complications and her hospitalization was over two weeks. Her husband had received a liver transplant four years earlier and was unable to stay in the hospital, so many of her friends volunteered to be there with Reneé every night. My parents and my three other sisters lived out of state and we were in constant contact with each other. One of my sisters flew in for a day and a half to be there when the doctor did rounds. I remember calling and talking with Reneé during that long hospitalization and she always had visitors.

Reneé started Intraperitoneal Chemo treatments in June 2005. Our family never could have imagined that when Reneé finished the chemo treatments, she would only have a year before the ovarian cancer would return in 2007. Later, I found out that in that year her CA125 had been increasing each month. From 2007, until two weeks before her death, Reneé was on constant chemo treatments including clinical trials. One of the clinical trials she participated in involved an oral drug and one day she got a phone call from the Oncology Nurse to stop taking the drug as women were having heart attacks and the clinical trial was being discontinued. Not living in the same state, I wanted to learn as much as I could about ovarian cancer treatments and drugs. Every time Reneé started a new chemo drug, I would start researching the drug. I learned more than I ever thought I would know about ovarian cancer chemo drugs. I brought up Avastin to Reneé when it started being in the news regarding ovarian cancer. When her doctor decided that it was time for Reneé to be on Avastin, I felt that I understood the side effects. Yet, we are never able to fully understand the effects of the chemo drugs on our loved ones. In July 2010, Reneé started chemo with Doxil, a big step for her because she loved to be out in the sun and drinking hot coffee. I will always remember in August 2010 talking to her one morning and her telling me she was drinking cold coffee and that it was OK.

Reneé never let her cancer define her or stop her from experiencing life. After Reneé was diagnosed with ovarian cancer we took three sister trips to Florida beaches. Reneé loved to sit out in the sun all day and we all would sit out with Renee all day, even though she did not have sisters who shared her love of the beach. November 2009, Reneé was excited that my sisters and parents were all going to go to Washington, D.C. That weekend we enjoyed being together and that Sunday we all competed in the Race to End Women's Cancer. In my office, I have the picture of Reneé going across the finish line holding our sister Jeanine's hand. Renee's doctor from OU was at the Race and Dr. Moore ran with my sister Janet as she could see the matching shirts we were all wearing. On the front of the teal shirt it said "Hope is Passion For What is Possible," and on the back of the shirt it said, "Live, Laugh and Love," with all four of our initials underneath. That shirt signified the love of all four sisters and reminded me of the strong bond we always had.

Reneé never wanted ovarian cancer to define her and never wanted anyone to feel bad for her because she had cancer. Being very private about having ovarian cancer, I will never forget when she was in Palliative Care at OU Medical Center and the nurse asked how long she had ovarian cancer. Reneé responded in a strong voice that she had ovarian cancer for five and ½ years. It touched my to heart to hear her response because when she was diagnosed, doctors told her that her life expectancy was 5 years. At the Race in D.C. in November 2009, I had met Dr. Mannel from OU Medical and he had told me Reneé was one of their longest Ovarian Cancer patients.

Reneé taught kindergarten from her diagnosis in 2005 until her final hospitalization in September 2010. The teachers at her school, Northern Hills Elementary in Edmond, Oklahoma supported her in so many ways. For the school pictures all the teachers wore teal one year. The teachers and school staff all wore teal yarn bracelets and took a picture with all of their hands together. When I look at the picture it reminds me how many people supported Reneé during her battle with ovarian cancer. Two weeks before her death she received the award for Northern Hills Elementary Teacher of The Year. The Northern Hills Principal and the Superintendent of Edmond Schools came to OU Medical Center to present Reneé with the award. I took pictures and Reneé had the biggest smile on her face even though she was seriously ill… she was thrilled to get the award.

The one thing that I learned from Renee's fight was that Ovarian Cancer changes not only the life of the patient, but also the life of the family and friends. Ovarian cancer is not a cancer that people talk about. Before Reneé was diagnosed, I admit that at age 49 all I knew was that the actress Gilda Radner had ovarian cancer. It was the cancer I knew that you did not want. In 2004 my neighbor's 80 year old mother was diagnosed and I remembered thinking at the time how sad, having no idea that in a year Reneé would be diagnosed.

In the past eleven years I have met many ovarian cancer survivors. I have been thankful that many have shared their journeys with me through e-mails, letters, phone calls, cards and personal visits. I always reached out to the families when one of these women passed away, be it attending the service or writing a letter to let them know their loved ones touched my life. Special angels who left a mark on my heart are Julene, Cecilia, Sharon, Benita, Nancy, Martha, Bekah, Audrey and Gay. Some of these women were friends of mine before they were diagnosed or I met them after their diagnosis. My college friend, Kim is a 10 year Ovarian Cancer Stage 3C Survivor. My dear friend Lucy called me the day after I returned from attending Renee's memorial service in Oklahoma to tell me her sister-in-law Martha age 50, had been diagnosed at stage 3C. I had tears in my eyes five years later when I sat in the pew at Martha's memorial service.

I continue to meet many ovarian cancer survivors and family members whose lives have been touched by ovarian cancer. These individuals encourage me to work hard to advocate for ovarian cancer research and awareness. I strongly believe in research for an early detection test for ovarian cancer and have been actively involved in raising funds for Colleen's Dream Foundation. I have advocated in D.C. on the Hill through the Ovarian Cancer Research Fund Alliance and encourage others to contact their elected representatives in D.C. about ovarian cancer issues. I have supported GOCA and The Ovarian Cancer Institute. I helped in 2008 with a billboard campaign in Atlanta through the National Ovarian Cancer Coalition. I always tell others that ovarian cancer is a cancer you need to be aware of and understand the symptoms. To those I meet who have lost family members, I always say we are the voice for our loved ones now in educating others about ovarian cancer and working for more research, especially an early detection test.

The end of June 2010 we took a family beach trip and one of the pictures that I will always cherish is of Reneé and my younger sister Jeanine standing by the Gulf of Mexico. I always will have my sister Renee in my heart as her love always will guide me as I speak out about ovarian cancer. Reneé Lobodinski Specht left this world on October 1, 2010, and she left her mark on the hearts of her family and friends.

Chapter 22

God Does Have a Plan

By Tammy Lucia
(Daughter-in-law of Jaye Lucia)

I remember in the mid-seventies when I was in middle school in Shreveport, Louisiana, my Mom told us our grandmother, her mother, had cancer. I think I was in 6th grade, and had never known anyone who had cancer, so I don't think I realized the magnitude of this news. About 6 months into her fight my mother took all four of her girls to Cincinnati to be close to her, so we could help and spend time with her. As a young girl I wasn't understanding why we were leaving our school, friends, and dad to go to a strange school away from all that was familiar "for a few months." My grandmother died that next year from "the cancer." I later found out it was ovarian cancer. At the time not knowing ovarian cancer would enter my life again later during my life.

Fast forward to February 2000, we were living in Columbus Ohio, Bruce was the President of the Kroger division at that time. We got a call from his oldest sister telling us that their Mom, Jaye had been diagnosed with stage 4 ovarian cancer. She was 79 years old and her prognosis was grim, it had spread close to her lungs. Now along with this news her oldest son Ray was battling ALS, and husband was very ill with many things, but primarily emphysema and she was his caregiver. But let me tell you something about Jaye Lucia, she was a fighter. Without any complaints she immediately started chemo. She has always had the best attitude and spiritual heart. After a few rounds of chemo she had surgery. I flew to Atlanta to take care of Dad Lucia while she was in the hospital. When we would visit her daily she always had every nurse on the floor in love with her, she was a genuinely sweet southern belle. After surgery she settled into a routine of chemo, and taking care of her husband.

In September of that year her son Ray lost his fight with ALS. It was so heartbreaking for the whole family but to watch both Mr. and Mrs. Lucia say goodbye to their son, there are no words. This is when I realized how incredibly strong and spiritual my mother-in-law really was. As a mother of two boys I'm not sure I could handle losing a child as well as she did, and with such grace and poise.

She said to me one day "God has a plan for all of us and I'm not to question him." She felt it was so important to share every possible memory of Ray to keep him in our thoughts, and help fight our grief, she was amazing.

As she said, "God does have a plan." In October we found out we were moving back to Atlanta. The boys and I moved back one week before Christmas 2000. I quickly settled us into our home, which strategically was a little over a mile from her house. When my boys were settled, I volunteered to take her to her chemo and appointments. Now let me clarify something, Bruce and I married when he left Atlanta. Other than some holidays and summer visits once a year I didn't know Mrs. Lucia that well. But with her chemo, doctor appointments, scans, and all that comes with the treatment of ovarian cancer, we spent a lot of time with Mrs. Lucia, and I feel blessed to have had all that time. We never went to any appointment without gifts for nurses, doctors, pharmacists, and other patients. She oozed sweetness.

Although her prognosis at the beginning was grim, her strength and faith prevailed. She went through two remissions followed by reoccurrences each time. Around spring of 2008 she once again started another round of chemo. In the eight years of her fight, this was the first time her little body could not endure the chemo. After two rounds she chose to stop chemo and live the rest of her time with as much enthusiasm as she had all her life.

In October of 2009, I was meeting a friend in Boston for a long weekend. Mrs. Lucia was so excited, she loved Boston. She shared many stories from when they lived in Massachusetts, during one of Mr. Lucia's assignments with the Air Force. As I arrived in Boston and turned on my phone the messages started, CALL HOME! I immediately called and Mrs. Lucia had taken an unexpected turn. With this news, I ready to turn around and go back home, she was not having it. I was to stay and enjoy my first visit to Boston, and bring home lots of pictures and stories. Against all my instincts I did what she wanted, and she was right, Boston was everything she said it would be.

When I returned on Sunday, the first thing my husband said was, "my Mom is waiting up to see you." We went straight there and I climbed into bed with her and told her all about my trip, and showed her the pictures she asked me to take. She was weak, but she made me feel so loved and I knew I had become as special to her as she was to me. Mrs. Jaye Lucia died two days later at the age of 88. She fought ovarian cancer with strength and faith for over nine years!! She never let it stop her from doing anything she wanted to do. Her faith never wavered. She did not let the disease define or rule her life, she lived every day to its fullest.

In honor of my grandmother, Dorothy Coffey and mother-in-law, Jaye Lucia I serve on the board of Georgia Ovarian Cancer Alliance. It was important for me to help others fighting and living with this disease.

Chapter 23

Love Had Nothing to Do With It

By Marty McAtee

My mother died of breast cancer in 1955 when I was 15. It had metastasized in her bones. As a result, I had regular mammograms and was consistent with my medical checkups. I later learned that there is no test to identify ovarian cancer.

My ovarian cancer symptoms were different from many others'. I experienced reoccurring bladder infections and an extreme loss of weight. I blamed the weight loss on the fact that I was in love with the man who is now my husband after living alone for 24 years. Then, in February of 2009, while we were vacationing in Florida, I had difficulty catching my breath while we were playing tennis. My normal endurance level was different. When we returned to Marietta, where we were living, Jerry took me to Urgent Care. The physician there told me I was a very sick lady and called 911 for an ambulance. I was transported immediately to Northside Hospital in Atlanta. After a series of tests, it was determined that I had pulmonary embolisms, and fluid in my lungs.

The admitting physician in the Emergency Room told me he thought I had ovarian cancer. That was the shock of my life. However, at the time, I was not aware of the number of cancer-related deaths from this horrible disease. I personally did not know of anyone who had it. I suppose if I thought I was going to get cancer, breast cancer would have been the one.

Fortunately, a gynecological oncologist was on call, and four days later I received my first chemotherapy treatment. Fluid was extracted from my abdomen and lungs and I was put on Coumadin for the blood clots. A filter was also inserted to prevent further blood clots from getting to my heart or lungs. I was diagnosed with Stage 4 Ovarian Cancer. I spent eleven days in the hospital at that time experiencing every test imaginable. After I established a primary care physician, I was released.

My doctor proceeded with several rounds of chemotherapy believing that shrinking the tumors was important prior to surgical removal. He was also seeing whether my body would react favorably to the chemo. Fortunately, on my 69th birthday in March of 2009, I was told that I would live. For one month I lived without knowing if I had a chance of survival or not.

During all of that time, I was also going weekly for tests to determine if the level of Coumadin was correct in my body. Also, I was losing my hair all over our house. Jerry took me into the bathroom and cut off all my hair while I cried.

In April of 2009, I had a complete hysterectomy along with what is called the HIPEC. It is a washing of the entire interior of one's body with chemotherapy. The nausea as a result of that was terrible -- worse than the pain from the surgery. All I knew was that whatever it took for me to live was worth it. That hospital stay lasted nine days. Both my daughter and my now step-daughter were there for the surgery and were crying when they saw me in the recovery room. If one can envision someone with no hair and tubes coming out everywhere that is what I must have looked like.

Then the rounds of chemo began. Of course, I didn't feel so great after each round. My physician prescribed six rounds consisting of 3 treatments per round. I asked him why and he told me that he had the best success with that number. My taste buds changed, and foods that I used to enjoy didn't taste good. Sometimes, all I felt like eating was soup or a grilled cheese sandwich.

When I came home from the hospital, I began walking. I decided if walking was what the doctors wanted you to do in the hospital, there must be a reason. Loving the outdoors, I began walking outside. The first day, I couldn't make it around the block where we lived. This was difficult to accept for someone who had been addicted to exercise all of my life. I used to run at least three miles five days a week along with playing tennis often. When I was working while I lived in Indianapolis, I was up at 5:00 a.m. and at the gym by 5:30. Eventually, I was able to walk one mile, then two and so forth. I now walk three miles several days a week along with playing tennis and golf. I am convinced that exercise is important for recovery.

During my recovery, I spent a great deal of time on the couch and became an avid Braves fan, although it has been difficult lately. It was helpful as I had always enjoyed baseball. Although I have always been an avid reader, I found that my concentration level was not what it once had been.

Because I had come here late in 2008, I had not had time to make many friends. Jerry was just about it in my life as far as friends go and that was difficult. It was a lonely time for me, I was in touch with friends in Indiana and Kentucky primarily on email, and the cards and notes I received were wonderful. I still have them. I also know that people all over the world were praying for me. The trip to the mailbox each day was usually a happy event. I send many notes and cards myself, as I know what they meant to me. My daughters who live all over the country came to see me, and my brother and sister-in-law visited as well.

When I completed my last chemo treatment, my physician referred me to a breast surgeon since I had tested positive to the BRCA1 and 2 tests. I had planned to return to Indiana, but Jerry asked me to marry him. The day after we were married in December of 2009, I was diagnosed with breast cancer, and six months later I had a lateral mastectomy and reconstructive surgery. That is a story for another day. My breast oncologist told me that she believed my physical condition was the reason I had survived.

I believe one's attitude about things helps a great deal when one is diagnosed with a disease from which you could die. Some people just give up, but during that month when I didn't know if I would live or die, I knew I wanted to live to see my grandchildren grow up, graduate from college and get married. I had a great deal to live for. However, I sometimes ask myself, why did I live and so many others do not.

I still have neuropathy in my feet, and what we who have had cancer refer to as "chemo brain". My age could have something to do with that. I play tennis and golf four or five days a week and I see my oncologist once a year. In September of 2016, it will be seven years for me. I am grateful for every day.

Chapter 24

Not a Way to Bring in The New Year

By Shetabia Morgan-Putmon

"Baby, my back is hurting me so bad", as I explained to my husband. He told me to come and lie down and rest. It was Christmas Eve and I was looking out the window, it was raining and I was debating if I was going to church. My back was aching so badly, I decided to go to bed. As I'm lying there, it starting stinging worst, like needles on my side. I put up with the pain until the 12th hour of Christmas Eve 2009, and finally I just woke my husband up and said, "honey I can't take this pain anymore, please take me to the emergency room!"

As we proceeded to leave out the house, we were arguing about what hospital was I going to, and he insisted on Emory. I had never been to Emory, and never thought my insurance would be taken by Emory, but he didn't care and was really adamant about going. As I'm lying in the bed in the emergency room, I noticed how bloated my stomach was and I kept telling my husband, I'm probably getting ready to get my cycle or I have a urinary tract infection.

The nurse came in and asked all kind of medical questions. The main ones were "Do you have kids? Are you trying to get pregnant?" I answered no and yes. Yes we are trying to get pregnant, but to have intercourse just wasn't feeling right. It felt like someone was ramming a stick inside of me, it was so painful. We also told the nurse we were going to get married that Monday after New Years' Day, which was January 4, 2010. So the nurse said, "That's wonderful and congratulations, but I'm going to have to take a CT scan to see what is going on." My husband and I looked at each other and said, "What is a CT scan?" The nurse explained that I would have to drink this white contrast, and then would have a dye injected into my body to see what was going on. She proceeds to say "It's not as painful as you think." We agreed to do it, we wanted to get back to trying to having a baby, both of us laughing.

The nurse wheeled me around to the CT scan area, I didn't have a worry in the world, just ready for them to give me something for my pain so I could go home. After the CT scan she rolled me back to the room and my husband and I started playing games and joking. We called my Mom because we were supposed to be at a family breakfast, I told my Mom I was in the emergency room, and not to worry, we would be leaving soon, but we wouldn't make the breakfast. She panicked and came to the hospital anyway.

The nurse returned with the results, it was heart wrenching. "Ms. Morgan you have two tumors on your ovaries, one the size of a grapefruit and the other one the size of an orange!" All of the conversation stopped between my Mom, husband and I…you could hear a pin drop. So I said, "Ok, remove the tumors so we can proceed to try to have kids." Then the nurse said, "Ms. Morgan you don't understand, after we remove the tumors which are causing you so much pain during intercourse, they will have to be tested to see if they are cancerous." I still said "Ok let's do it because we are getting married on Monday, and we want some kids." Then the low blow came, she took the breath right out of our bodies. "Ms. Morgan you won't be able to have kids!" There was a dead silence. Tears were rolling down me and my husband's face. She said I would need a total hysterectomy immediately, and she sent me to the best gynecologic oncologist at Emory who was a specialist in cancer patient care.

Before I go on, let me tell you about my husband Terrell. We met at my best friends' birthday party which was on a Monday, January 22, 2009. We hit it off so well it was like a breath of fresh air for the both of us. We had been in crazy relationships previously, and it was just good to meet someone who was at the same level in life as you are. Our first date lasted approximately 11hrs straight, just talking about anything and everything. Oh, my heart was beating so fast because I had just gotten out of a previous relationship with this abusive guy, but the guy kept lingering around like a stray cat. I was so afraid that Terrell would not want to have anything to do with my drama, until I had closed that chapter of my life.

Finally, I had to get a restraining order against the ex-boyfriend, and had him locked up in order for him to leave me alone. I was so blessed to have Terrell by my side, but it was up to me to call the police, just so he would know that I was sincere about moving on, and ending that chapter of my relationship with the devil. After that, things went smoothly with Terrell and I, and we saw each other every day when I got off work. We were inseparable. We dated for about a year and he started talking about marrying me. I was so nervous because I would have never thought I would be getting married after being in an abusive relationship.

His Mom told him he was moving too fast and my mother said the same thing. We both explained that we had been through so many relationships, and we were not getting any younger and we both knew what exactly what we wanted. He was my soul mate, best friend, and confidant. It seems like we were meant to be. We both knew God put us together for a reason. He was 100% in my corner about everything. He proposed to me in November of 2009. We set the date to be married on January 4, 2010. We didn't want a wedding, but surely a big reception.

We started planning for the reception in December of 2009. By the end of December of 2009, New Year's Eve to be exact, that is when I experienced the pain on my side and in my back, which brings us back to the emergency room at Emory. I was so scared of losing Terrell, because we were just told we couldn't have kids, and I have to have a hysterectomy, plus I had to have these tumors removed and they may be cancerous.

Terrell was by my side the entire time, not even mentioning he was going to leave me. We did discuss the courthouse, and we both agreed on that Monday, January 4th would be the day. I was so happy and scared at the same time, knowing my life was getting ready to change, meaning I might have cancer and my last name won't be the same. It was a huge step for the both of us.

The day arrived and we got married, then went onto the doctor's office to set up the date for my surgery. The doctor couldn't believe that we had just gotten married. My husband had gotten over the fact that we couldn't have kids, just as long as I was healthy. They performed the surgery and I was diagnosed with Ovarian Cancer Stage IIIc. It was silent in the room, and I kept seeing faces of disbelief. I kept asking everybody "Why are you looking like that?" Then the doctor came in.

It still didn't sink in when I was at the hospital until the doctors said I had to do chemotherapy. Then it hit me. The room was dark, and all I could think about, was I just got married to the soulmate of my life, please God don't take him away from me. I cried and prayed at the same time because I knew my life would never be the same. I have been fighting ovarian cancer since 2010, been in remission for one year in 2011, then it came back. Then I beat it again in 2012. It came back in 2013. I was in remission for 6 months and now I'm fighting as I am writing my story. I never even heard of Ovarian Cancer, let alone knew the symptoms. I do know that my grandmother passed away from Ovarian Cancer at the age of 84.

I wasn't aware of the BRCA gene test. If I had known what I know now, I probably would have saved my own life, literally! I did get my regular Pap smear checkups. I knew when I dropped the ball, but I didn't have the heart to tell my parents. I was too cheap to pay the $300 for the ultrasound when I was in so much pain from my side. Yep, that's what my OB/GYN wanted: $300.00. I knew it was my fault and I had to speak up fast.

Unexpectedly on the night I was in the hospital trying to come up with a plan to tell my Mom, I see this tall guy with pearly white teeth walk in my room. It was my uncle, my Mom's brother. I was crying so badly and he asked me what was wrong? I told him the situation regarding the $300, and how I was too cheap to pay for an ultrasound, and the cancer could have been prevented. Also, I

207

told him "my Mom is going to call the OB/GYN and let her know that legal action for her negligence will be brought against her." I told my uncle it wasn't the doctor's fault, it was my fault and I don't have the guts to tell my Mom. So he agreed to tell her and told me everything is going to be okay.

I asked my uncle, "Why did it have to be me to get cancer?" He responded, "Why not you?" You are one of His soldiers on the battlefield, and He knows who can fight and be a winner." That stuck with me until this very day, as I often keep asking the question "Why me?" So I always remember because I am a soldier for the Lord. I won't give up this fight because I'm afraid of disappointing God. He has a huge purpose for me being on this earth, and I'm going to enjoy every minute of it. My motto is: ALWAYS MAKE IT COUNT! Don't Judge UNTIL you know my story!

LADIES, LADIES, LADIES...PLEASE GET CHECKED OUT. DO NOT LET $300.00 COME BETWEEN YOU AND YOUR HEALTH. IF I WOULD HAVE GOTTEN THE ULTRASOUND...WOULDA, SHOULDA, COULDA.......GO GET CHECKED!!

Chapter 25

Ovarian Cancer Through the Eyes of a Son

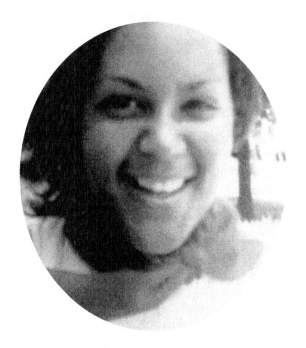

By Ray Muhammad
(Son of Frances Elaine Sanders)

This is the story of Frances Elaine Sanders, born September 21, 1950 from a surviving son's perspective. Growing up in Atlanta, Elaine was known for her high intelligence, quick wit and penchant for light hearted mischief. One of her legendary pranks as a child was to call cab after cab to her neighbor's house, and watch as they blew their horns while the neighbor came out to shoo them away. Her love of laughter was passed on to her children. Elaine was tall, beautiful and a very talented pianist.

Elaine and her husband Albert had three children: a son Ray followed by twin girls, Tiffanie and Tracie. She had Ray at seventeen years of age, and the closeness in age also helped make them closer to one another. She was a very proud and dedicated mother, investing heavily in her children, their education and overall maintenance and well-being.

Elaine was also very influential to young people in her community. She was a substitute teacher and also contributed by teaching the arts to young children in her locale. Elaine was a proprietor, owning Perspective 21, a school of performing arts. This studio taught ballet, gymnastics, piano, and martial arts. Several of her former students went on to performing arts high schools, earned college scholarships and became professional performers. Even today, her former students frequently point to her as a motivating source of their accomplishments in life.

In 1984 at the age of 34, Elaine Sanders was diagnosed with ovarian cancer. She did not tell many people about this newly discovered disease and refused to let it control her life. Elaine went to chemotherapy but was unhappy, the disease did not allow her to continue to care for her family as she had done in the past. After several sessions of therapy, she decided she would not go back. Cancer would continue to take a toll on Elaine physically, but never would it rob her of her dignity, spirit of determination, sense of humor, or her resolve to be a great caregiver to her biological children and extended circle of children.

Elaine's journey over the next year became a very challenging journey. One which she undertook with class and strength that affected and served as inspiration to everyone who witnessed it. She prepared her family for what was to come as best she could. Doing so without ever allowing anyone to be depressed or sad about what was now a reality for her and us.

At one point in 1985, I recall my mother being hospitalized. It is possible she had surgery but she explained the visit as nothing serious. When it was time for her release, my father did not drive to pick her up so she called and had me to bring my sisters. Although, it was tough for me to handle, Elaine was determined that this was a day to celebrate. We went to IHOP, one of her favorite restaurants and enjoyed breakfast with family. This was just one of several Moments that would be permanently etched in my memory which exemplified what a classy woman Elaine was.

Because of her belief that she was the protector over her children, Elaine didn't reveal the extent of her disease to us. She prepared my sisters and me without us even knowing, consciously taking steps to isolate us from her suffering. We now recall fondly how she would let my sisters help choose the hospital she would stay when there was a choice. She had become such a frequent visitor, my sisters had a ranking based on which facility had the best cafeteria. She made them focus on the delightful cuisine as opposed to her worsening condition. She also worked to provide comfort for us after she would be gone, by writing special letters to each of her children.

My mother was concerned how I would handle her death. I was a seventeen-year-old freshman at Florida State University, away from

211

her for the first time and she did not want to see me fail. I had suggested staying home because I could tell she was sick, for one because the living room was now her bedroom because she could no longer climb our stairs. She insisted I go to college as planned and would hear nothing of me delaying my start. As she put me on this path, she put a plan into action to ensure my mental health and focus when she was gone. My twin sisters had and would have one another but she feared I would have no one.

My mother was well liked by all of my friends. In fact, I can remember being a bit "jealous" while other friends borrowed her privately for advice on serious situations they faced. So when she came to them, they were eager to respond. My mother met with my closest friends and asked them to promise to look out for me, and be there for me so I would not give up on life. It would be years before I would have any idea of these meetings which is another testimony of their love for her. My friends loved and respected her so much they would not break her confidence in them, even for me.

Entering the fall of 1985, there were Momentous Moments for Elaine. My mother witnessed Tiffanie and Tracie graduate from middle school, and Tracie won Ms. Ninth Grade at her high school. She was alive to see me go off to college after graduating high school and she celebrated her thirty-fifth birthday. When I came home for that celebration, she was thinner and looked a little tired but she was in great spirit. We had a party for her birthday and visited Red Lobster.

I assume everyone had possibly come to realize just how serious her condition was, so the family was supportive. My mother was still determined to be "Mommy." She washed my clothes against my objection and cooked. She was determined to hear all about college and make sure I was well, as she did the same every day for my sisters. At that time, I was still encouraging her to "beat cancer" and she assured me she would, knowing I was in denial of what was to come.

In October 1985, I visited my mother once again. She seemed a little weaker, her skin a little darker, but she still "fought" me, taking my laundry basket as I was about to wash my clothes during my visit. I was beginning to realize this didn't look good and she encouraged me to be as normal as possible. She didn't allow me to sit around the house with her all weekend, encouraging me to visit friends. On a phone call in late October, I could hear in her voice the toll cancer was taking on her. I finally asked how SHE was feeling as opposed to my usual motivational speech to kick cancer's butt. She sighed and said, "well Ray, I'm just tired". That was the first time I heard her say that; I told her that if she was tired, she should go rest and we would be fine.

The weekend of November 8, 1985 would be the last time I spoke with my Mom or saw her. She had been hospitalized and was deteriorating rapidly when I arrived for my weekend visit. She was as delightful as ever when I saw her; she looked like a little girl. She was still very polite and concerned about everyone but herself, but by Sunday she was slipping in and out of consciousness.

I was preparing to go back to school and hugged my mother in her bed. She asked if I was leaving and I said "yes" as I kissed her. She said, "well when you come back, I will be" and she fell asleep I guess. I was so afraid I asked "you will be what? You will be what?" but she didn't respond. I hugged everyone and left the room in tears. As I began walking away, they yelled that my mother was calling for me. I returned and she picked up as if she had never stopped, "I'll be here" was what she said. She was then, she is now; no matter where my sisters and I go.

Chapter 26

It's a Whole New World

By Bryan Ray
(Husband of Jessica Ray)

My name is Bryan Ray. I had the cookie cutter life, the American dream! I married my high school sweetheart Jessica Morey after we both graduated from Pebblebrook High School in Cobb County Georgia. We had a wonderful wedding attending by all of our family and friends. Our favorite song during our wedding was "It's a whole new world", it was sung by two of our closest friends and everyone loved it. Especially Jess. We were on top of the world.

Shortly after our wedding we had a beautiful healthy baby girl that we named Savannah Nicole Ray in March of 1999. She was such a wonderful baby. In February of 2002, we had another healthy baby, this time a handsome little boy, Alexander Justus Ray! It was truly everything a man could ask for in a loving wife, 2 healthy kids and even fantastic in-laws.

After Alex was born we decided that our family was complete. Jess made an appointment and went in to get an IUD device as a method of birth control. Shortly after she got the IUD, she starting having some discomfort. So she made an appointment with her OB/GYN to get checked out.

As most things in life I just thought, oh, it's nothing, she will get an antibiotic and it will be fine. However, while at work I got a call from Jess, and the first time I heard her breathe into the phone I knew something wasn't right. I immediately regretted not going to the appointment with her. She told me that her doctor had found something, but it was "probably nothing" but he wanted to check it out. After some tests and scans there was a mass detected. Two words that put your world on tilt, mass and detected. We both still told ourselves that it was nothing and everything would be fine. Nothing could happen to us, the all American family!

The surgery was scheduled shortly after at Cobb Hospital in December of 2003, the surgeon was Dr. Hines. I had never met Dr. Hines, but I had heard he was the best! We arrived very early the morning of her surgery along with many of our family members. We have a great deal of love between our two families. Everyone was there to hear the usual, the surgery went well, and she did great, she will be better soon, that sort of thing.

We got an update from the lady at the desk after several hours and she seemed to have good news. The surgery was over and everything went well. Everyone breathed a sigh of relief. Dr. Hines came out and asked Jessica's mother Cindy and I to come behind a small partition with him. The details of that conversation were a little fuzzy, but I remember him telling us that it was not good news and that he thought she had Ovarian Cancer and needed treatment. Somehow I recall him saying that it was squamous cell cancer of a dermoid cyst. I couldn't really tell you what that is, but I knew it meant my family was in for a tough fight.

That was probably the worst night of not only my life but most everyone that was in that waiting room along with Jess and her parents. We had the overwhelming task of knowing what had been found while Jess rested peacefully in her room. We waited for her to wake up so we could deliver this horrible and heartbreaking news. I am so thankful for my family and friends support that night, it was awful and we could not have endured it alone.

Those of you that knew Jess knew how positive and bubbly she was, so while the news upset her after a few minutes of tears and worry she was ready to fight. To fight for Savannah and Alex, to fight for her parents Tom and Cindy, and to fight for herself. She had her whole life ahead of her and she was not ready to give up.

The next 15 months was hell. I think 4 or 5 more surgeries along with 3-4 different types of chemotherapy, and it seemed like nothing was working. I remember one visit with Dr. Hines, when we went in after a scan and while Dr. Hines was always so positive and always wearing a smile his words hit us like a ton of bricks.

"This is not a good turn of events". Dr. Hines had a way with words, and if there was any silver lining he would have found it. So when he delivered such a simple and direct sentence we knew it was bad.

He basically told us that it was time to decide to keep fighting and prolong the pain, or just stop treatment and enjoy the best quality of life for the time we all had left together. Let me tell you, this is not a fun conversation to have with someone you love.

I left the decision 100% up to Jess, as I had no idea what she was going through physically. I could see the pain and we talked about everything, and how I knew how hard it was as a caregiver, I could not image how she felt. She made what I believe was the right decision, and decided to come home and be with her family for as much time as she could.

Let me stop and tell you about our family for a second, my parents Claude and Sheila Ray cared for the kids like they were their own. My dad and brother-in-law, Kyle Phillips came over and in one day built a ramp for our 20ft high patio so we could roll a wheel chair down it. My sister Sandy helped me day and night, and basically became a nurse alongside me. Jessica's parents Tom and Cindy traveled tirelessly, and would stay overnight to help take care of her and the kids. We basically made a hospital room in one of the kid's room at our house.

The crazy thing is that Jess never played the victim, she stayed strong and positive and kept loving everyone, and continued to make everyone laugh. I don't know how anyone in her condition can do that, but if anyone could it was Jess.

She stayed mobile and fought hard for a while, we celebrated Alex's 2nd birthday on February 13, 2004. It was almost like she was waiting for that milestone, because less than a week later I had to make the impossible decision of moving her to hospice.

It really gets foggy at this point, almost like it wasn't really happening. I think she was in hospice maybe 36 hours or so. I remember my sister was in the room with me, and Jess was really struggling for life. Sandy and I walked outside the room on a small back patio and I began to weep. I had my head on Sandy's shoulder and I told her that it was ok for Jess to let go, as I looked over her shoulder I watched Jess take a very peaceful deep last breath, and then she was gone. This may sound made up, but that is exactly the way it happened. Even though I knew it was coming the pain was more than I could have ever imagined.

Through all of this there was one thing that I regret, the night that Jess passed I called my parents who were at home watching Savannah and Alex. I asked Mom to tell them what had happened. I deeply regret that, I should not have put her in that position but I didn't know if I could handle it.

That night was tough of course, but it was not as tough as the night of her surgery at Cobb Hospital. You may ask why, my answer is that I knew when she passed away that her fight was over, the pain was gone and she was now in heaven.

Just to let you know how special Jess was to anyone she met, I remember at the funeral home the night before she was buried, I stood by her casket and shook hands and gave out hugs to hundreds of people. I will admit I can't tell you who all was there as it was a surreal feeling. However, I remember seeing a line of people probably 30 yards long that went out of the front door of the funeral home.

I definitely recall one person that night, late in the evening when most people were gone, I recognized Dr. Hines walking up. He was in his scrubs and even still had his surgeon cap on his head. He approached me with tears in his eyes, and apologized for the way he was dressed. I gave him a huge hug, and thanked him for everything he did for Jess. He took it personal that we all lost that battle. He was a doctor that genuinely cared about his patients, or at least he cared about Jess. He prayed with us many times and was always positive but honest with us. I took that as the biggest compliment in the world that he would drive out to the funeral home after who knows how many hours of surgery, just to pay his respects to Jessica. I think that speaks for itself.

The following day at the funeral our family and friends all gathered at Ephesus Baptist church in Winston, Ga. I am not sure why, but I was determined to get up and speak during the service. Again, I don't remember exactly what I said, but I know the message was to convey that tomorrow is not a guarantee and live every day like it is your last. I urged everyone to go home and hug their wife, mother or father, and tell them how much they love them! The same song that was played at our wedding "It's a whole new world" was also played. While a completely different meaning, still a perfect choice.

The service concluded inside the church, and we moved to the burial site outside the church. As everyone gathered around the burial site I recall the immense noise of frogs croaking in the woods that surround the cemetery. Like magic when Rev. Billy Godwin started to speak every single frog was silent. I couldn't help but smile. It was like this day was her peaceful day.

After the ceremony was over I shook hundreds of hands again, and received many loving hugs. I still didn't seem real. Alex was running around full of life and Savannah was smiling like she always does. I realized then that it was up to me to make sure that our kids would get to see and do everything that Jess wanted them too. My outlook on life is now, if you want to go somewhere, go!

If you want to do something, do it! If you want to buy something, buy it! You are not guaranteed tomorrow!

I see Jess in Savannah and Alex from time to time and it makes me smile. Jessica's parents are still 100% a part of Savannah and Alex's life, and love them more than ever. It makes me so happy to see them together.

I have remarried to a wonderful lady named Sara, and we now have a total of 4 kids. Our parents along with Tom and Cindy are really one big family and support system that will always make sure that our children will have everything they need to succeed in life.

We have all put on a few fundraisers in Jessica's honor and I served as a board member on the Georgia Ovarian Cancer Alliance for 2+ years. While the 4 kids have kept me too busy to stay on the board, we are ALL still heavily involved with GOCA and are committed to raising awareness about the deadly disease of Ovarian Cancer. We will keep fighting until we find a cure!

Chapter 27

I Am to Young to Have Ovarian Cancer

By Cindy Reynolds

I can't recall if I have ever shared my story in detail outside of the doctor's office or a Survivors Teaching Students session. Over the years I have started to provide the cliff note version because quite frankly, it's not something I like to re-live. The memories ignite so much emotion, both good and bad.

I moved back home from my first year at college. I remember coming down the steps at my parent's house and my neck was hurting. I had my hand on my neck and my Mom asked me what was wrong. I told her my neck hurt and as I moved my hand I could see the horror in her face. I had a golf ball sized lump on my neck and she made me go to the doctor immediately.

I had to get a biopsy on the lump (outpatient surgery) that left a scar on the side of my neck. My first battle wound. The morning we had the follow up appointment for the results, things were off. My Mom was very quiet and she wasn't herself. So I called my dad at work and asked him to tell me what was going on. He was reluctant at first, but I told him "I know it's not good" and I needed to know right then.

"Cindy, you have cancer." ….then silence.

At 19 years old, you truly believe you can conquer the world. When my dad told me they found cancer, I said I'm going to be ok, but I need to take care of Mom. My older sister died of cancer when she was 6. My parents had already lost 1 child and that is what I saw on my Mom's face that morning. She was in so much pain and so fearful. I didn't tell her I knew, I just put a smile on my face and tried to make her smile. We went into the doctor's office and she was trying to be so strong. We got called back to speak with the doctor and he started talking. It was too much, I couldn't bear to see her get this news so I stopped the doctor and turned to my Mom and said "Mom, I know that I have cancer, but I'm going to be ok. I'm not my sister and I'm strong enough to deal with this."

She started crying and I calmed her down and asked her to step outside of the room so that I could speak with the doctor on my own. That may seem strange, but I didn't want my Mom to re-live the pain of hearing her child has cancer.

In October 1997, I was diagnosed with Stage 4 Thyroid Cancer, cancer I had from my thyroid to my shoulder. I had a complete thyroidectomy and quite a bit of lymph nodes removed throughout my neck and shoulder. I was left with my second battle wound that stretched across the bottom of my neck and no feeling in my left shoulder. The surgery was followed by a high dose of radioactive iodine and close monitoring. Being so young, I really didn't know much about what a thyroid was or the importance of thyroid medicine. I took my medicine as prescribed, went to my doctor's appointments, got my scans, and occasionally I took my calcium which never gave me any problems.

I always struggled with my weight and the lack of a thyroid didn't help. In 2007 though, I was at the peak of my health working out twice a day. I lead a very social life in a motorcycle club, got a promotion at work, and started working nights. Life was as it should be in your 20s. Fun! I decided to switch my pharmacy to a location closer and somehow my thyroid medicine was switched as well. Basically it was just changed to a different generic version. Over the next year, my health drastically declined. I thought I was just getting use to the night shift, but later realized that wasn't it. I could no longer get on a motorcycle because riding 1 mile would leave me exhausted. I could no longer work out because I just didn't have the energy. I was physically drained, but I couldn't sleep. If I got 4 hours of sleep it was a good day.

I went to my endocrinologist for a check-up. Shared how I was feeling and the issues I was having. When my lab work came back my TSH was around 48 (normal range is 0.4 – 4.0). Basically the thyroid medicine I took for the last 6 months wasn't working, the doctor immediately put me on the brand version (Synthroid) and over the course of a few months my labs returned to a normal range.

Great! My labs are normal, but I still felt the same. On top of that, in a 2-month span I gained 40 pounds, anyone who has ever suddenly gained weight like this understands the strain it puts on your body. You are suddenly carrying around 40 extra pounds, your body didn't even get to adjust so its hard to breathe and move in general, let alone how it makes you feel about yourself. My endocrinologist had no answer for me, just that I should be fine and that he saw nothing wrong.

At this point you are probably wondering where the ovarian cancer comes in. Well...this is the story. Keep reading!

I started to see holistic doctors, naturopaths and doing a lot of research. I found a doctor who was about an hour from my house. He looked over my labs and diagnosed me with adrenal fatigue and advised I had reverse-T3. Adrenal what? Reverse what?

Adrenal fatigue is a term used in alternative medicine – you will not hear your in-network doctor use this term. The out-of-network docs use saliva tests that test the cortisol levels you are producing. The theory behind it is that the adrenals get fatigued and cannot produce/manage your cortisol appropriately. In a circadian cortisol schedule, your cortisol starts to rise around 6am to wake you up and get you moving. It continues to get higher and sometime after noon it will start to slowly decline. By the time it is time for you to go to bed, your cortisol should be at the lowest level so that you can sleep. For me, my cortisol did not rise. I was just always at that low level. Reverse T3 blocks the thyroid receptor and causes the symptoms of hypothyroidism. It elevates during times of stress and illness and was the root cause of many of my symptoms. As a result of my high reverse T3 and adrenal fatigue, I was changed to Armour Thyroid and put on multiple supplements. Finally I started getting some relief. I was able to sleep again and was getting some energy back. Yay!

So I started being able to function as a normal human being again. I should clarify that when I mean function as a normal human being, I mean getting back to myself. I am an introvert by nature so while I shared my health issues at times with friends it wasn't something I tried to show. I did my best to conceal what I was going through as many people with chronic health issues do. I used all my energy at work, ensuring I stayed focus and did my best to lead my team without bringing my personal issues into the workplace. I don't think it was until one of my friends stayed overnight at my house that someone truly understood I wasn't exaggerating about not sleeping.

So it's 2009 and I'm feeling better, but I still felt off. One of my best friends was pregnant and she was sharing her symptoms, mainly the frequent need to go to the restroom. Oddly enough, I was going to the restroom just as much! We joked that I was having pregnancy sympathy pain for her and I just thought I was drinking too much water. If that wasn't enough, I was having sharp pains under the right side of my rib cage. I went to the doctor numerous times and they finally ordered a HIDA scan. The tracer couldn't go past my gallbladder and due to a blocked bile duct I had emergency surgery to have my gallbladder removed. At least that got taken care of!

Throughout the years I was seeing a chiropractor at the time, Dr. Gail. What a wonderful woman! She was always so caring and understanding and although she was my chiropractor she would help me research information. She was following me closely and when I kept saying I was having certain symptoms she asked if I wanted her to order some labs that she had just started offering. At this point, I was willing to try anything! The labs measured all types of hormones, which I was unable to get any doctor to even think about doing.

My labs came back and my thyroid (TSH) was perfect, but my other hormones were all over the map. I will never forget looking at the results. Not only did it give results, but it gave possible causes for the levels. Under one of my tests there was a possible cause of an ovarian cyst. I started there since I had felt some bloating recently.

I went to my gynecologist, had my annual pap and she felt something in my abdomen. She ordered an ultrasound and there it was, a huge ovarian cyst. It was so huge, the lady performing the ultrasound asked me to empty my bladder again because she thought it was a full bladder. Through the ultrasound they could tell it was a complex cyst. My gynecologist suggested I take birth control pills to try to shrink the cyst and then come back to see her. Um… ok… really?

Thank God for the Internet! I googled the results and decided to go get a 2nd opinion. Same results, but this next gynecologist ordered tumor markers including the CA-125 test. The CA-125 came back in the 30s, I had no idea what this meant. She then referred me to a Gynecologic Oncologist. Whether it was possibly cancer or not, the cyst was so large she felt it was best for a specialist to remove it. I went to get a 3rd opinion and was told the same thing.

On to meet the gynecologic oncologist! By now I have looked up CA-125 and ovarian cancer was mentioned here or there. When I got to the Gyn-Onc, he advised I could rest assure that it was not Ovarian Cancer because it does not affect women my age. Great!

I had surgery scheduled in June 2010, the cyst was so large that they had to remove my left ovary which was completely surrounded by it. During the surgery they perform a surgical pathology to ensure there isn't something in the tissue that they may need to look at.

During my surgery the pathology came back as borderline ovarian cancer, so out went the cyst (which we will now call a tumor), my appendix, some lymph nodes, and some of my omentum. I woke up and was told about the borderline results and that they had sent off the tissue for a final pathology report which I would get in a few weeks. The tumor originally measured about 16cm, but when removed and laid out flat it was over 20cm! Centimeters…that is not a typo. The frequent urination that I was having was a result of the tumor constantly pressing on my bladder.

Wait, what happened to me being too young for ovarian cancer?! I'm going to need a refund Doc.

So I got a call on July 23, 2010 from the Gyn-Onc's nurse asking me to come into the office on Monday. This call was familiar or at least the tone of the call took me back to 1997. I didn't tell anyone I got the call, although the nurse kept telling me to bring someone with me. When I showed up by myself on Monday, July 26th the nurse and doctor asked if I wanted to call anyone. At this point, I am only thinking "just tell me already" so I can deal with this. So I got taken into a room again with the Gyn-Onc and nurse and it happened again…

"Cindy, you have Ovarian Cancer"…silence

The silence after you are told you have cancer is imaginary; the reality is the doctor/nurse/whomever is apologizing for the diagnosis. They are pumping you full of information and handing you folders with information, they have this look on their face…sympathy maybe? You can never be prepared to hear you have cancer. I knew walking into the doctor's office, but it doesn't become real until you sit face to face with the doctor and hear it come out of his mouth. It may just be hope that whatever you are going to be told will not be what you fear the most. In the Moment the doctor says you have cancer your hope balloon gets popped. Silence…the doctor was still talking, but I heard nothing except my internal thoughts, hopes, and dreams.

I thought I was too young? What about kids? Will I ever get married? What about my hair? What about my Mom? My dad? My brother? What about my friends? What about my job? Why is this happening again? What did I do? How will I get through this? What if I don't make it through?

Once the doctor handed me a binder and went over my treatment options, I left the office in complete shock. I went home and I cried. I struggled with how to break the news to my friends and family. I remember calling my Mom and telling her, she was devastated and she cried, but she knew I could beat it. I still couldn't talk, I didn't know what to do so I literally sent a text to my friends and told them I had cancer. I couldn't bring myself to speak it again because of how difficult it was to tell my family.

Chapter 28

Love at First Sight

By Christopher W. Seely
(Husband of Teri Seely)

My introduction to ovarian cancer began on my 20th anniversary. Teri and I disembarked for England in April of 2002 for London to begin our third decade together. We spent the night in London, then visited my aunt and uncle who had been living in England for the past 25 years. They suggested that since we had plans to visit the Cornwall coast that we walk some of the trails that are all over England. It was during our walks that Teri began to experience pain in her abdomen. Nothing she could put her finger on, just general pain and extreme discomfort. I, of course, just thought it was her (and mine, for that matter) lack of being in shape and told her we would both get better the more we walked. Prior to our trip, Teri had noticed a lump on the right side of her abdomen. She had seen a doctor about it and he told her it was most likely a small hernia, but nothing to be concerned about.

Upon our return, she went to a gynecologist, who just so happened to be a GYN/oncologist. When she mentioned the pain she experienced on our trip, he did an ultrasound. The interpretation of that procedure was that she had some fibroids, but again, nothing to worry about. We then discussed that since her "plumbing" was not working as well as it should, that perhaps she should have a hysterectomy. She was 46 and we had not planned to have any more children and agreed that it would be best to have the operation. It was scheduled for late August and it turned out to be the worst day of our lives.

We arrived at St. Joseph's hospital in Atlanta at 7am for the 9am procedure. The doctor said they should be finished by 10am, perhaps 11 at the latest. I waited in the lobby/waiting area. Ten o'clock came and went. So did 11, then noon. I inquired, but was told that she was in the operating room. 1, 2, and 3 o'clock all passed. More inquires, same response. I am now about to panic. 4 o'clock – still no word and by now all the people waiting had their loved ones' doctors come into the waiting area and inform them that their operations went well and they should be able to see them shortly. By 5, I was the only one there. The doctor finally came and with him was another doctor. I got up, went to him, but he held me off, and asked the receptionist for the key to the consultation room. I was informed that Teri had a large tumor on her left ovary, which was successfully removed. However, there was another tumor on her pancreas (that lump that was a hernia) and it could not be removed because it was too involved. One cannot live without a pancreas. I was also informed by the other surgeon that he was brought in to reconstruct her stomach and intestines since the tumor on her ovary had invaded those organs as well. Thus began the last year that Teri and I would spend together.

We spent the next two weeks in the hospital. I slept in her room and we consulted with the doctors on what would happen next: Chemo every 3 weeks for a few months. I was very fortunate in that Teri's mother was there every day, and her two best friends were present and willing and able to care for our boys and dogs while we were in the hospital. I was also fortunate in that my employer, American Airlines, told me to stay home and take care Teri, at least for now. We left the hospital, came home to our boys and puppies and prepared for the chemo sessions. Of course, Teri was still recovering from the hysterectomy and re-arranging of her internal organs. We were scared, but hopeful—and very, very tired.

The chemo started several weeks later in September, just before her 47th birthday. I stayed out of work until a week or so after the 1st session. In the meantime, we consulted another oncologist for a second opinion, whom did not offer an alternative treatment plan so we prepared for the chemo: cut her hair very, very short and did lots of Internet searches.

The first session was not too bad. She handled it well and since her mother was close, I went back to work. A side note here, in that I am an airline pilot, commuting to St. Louis, MO for my trips, which typically lasted 3-4 days. It was very helpful to have Teri's Mom close, as well as her friends. Teri did manage to return to "normal" home life a week or so after the chemo sessions, raising our boys and taking care of all the things one normally does. She wanted to have a regular routine, despite all.

Over the course of the next few months, I would stay home for her chemo sessions, then return to my schedule of 3-4 days at home, 3-4 days away flying. I worried all the time, but she was the calming one until the chemo took its toll and we ended up in the emergency room. It does amaze me how long it takes when you show up at an emergency room with a cancer patient, obviously in distress, for someone to actually do something. Her blood counts were way down and she needed a transfusion. She ended up getting admitted to the hospital for several days. I thought I was going to lose her right then and there, but she did recover and was sent home.

The first chemo did nothing, but we did make it to Christmas and through the winter. Her tumor was growing rather than shrinking, so back to the doctor to discuss a new course of treatment. We started a new regiment with a new chemo formula. She did not tolerate this chemo as well as the prior one. It really took a toll, and we ended in the emergency room several times for blood transfusions and the accompanying hospital stays. The stress was building and her tumor was still growing, so much so that occasionally it would breach the scar from her hysterectomy operation. The doctor re-stitched her stomach and I became proficient in wound care. So, not only was the tumor still growing, the chemo was taking its toll and she was now starting to bleed constantly. As the surgeon who did the stomach repair stated "your tumor started out as a baseball, it has grown into a softball and is now approaching a cantaloupe." I was rapidly losing hope, but Teri was still holding out. I kept up with her spirits and did not tell her my feelings.

We celebrated our 21st wedding anniversary in April. It was a subdued event, but still, I was joyful. 21 years with a lady I fell in love with at first sight. We met in Warner Robins, GA, her hometown though she had moved to Atlanta. I was living there, having just begun my airline career with a small regional airline. The day we met, we never looked back. We both knew we would be together for the rest of our lives.

In June, we took a trip to Vermont to celebrate my aunt and uncle's 50th wedding anniversary – the same aunt who lived in England. While there, Teri got very weak and her tumor was beginning to breach her abdomen. She thought it was just her stiches coming loose, but I knew better. I had to change her bandage daily, sometimes twice a day. We almost went to Dartmouth-Hitchcock Hospital in New Hampshire, but held off and made it back home.

I think now Teri knew things where not going to improve. July came and she entered the hospice program. I took a leave from work to be with her full time. We went to our house in Florida, a house we built and she loved dearly. I really think she wanted to die there, but instead got a second wind, though we did stay there over 3 weeks, we were back home in August. She was losing weight rapidly and it was difficult to see her in this condition. My beautiful Southern Lady was reduced to a staved skeleton with a basketball in her belly that refused to stop growing. She was in pain constantly, but the morphine that the hospice nurses gave her helped. I could no longer sleep in our bed next to her because of the breaching tumor and the need to change her dressing every few hours. I won't go into the details, but it was a mess that needed constant attention. I slept on the floor and was glad to at least be that close.

She passed away the last week of August. I refuse to remember the actual date. It is not important. She was born on September 23, 1955. She died at the age of 47, a month before her 48th birthday. She is gone, but she is still with me. Always will be, for rest of my life.

Footnote:

Being the caregiver is tough, very tough. You have to be there, you want to do things to help, but feel helpless because most of the time there is nothing you can do. It is very frustrating and sad. Your life changes as much as hers. Though you don't feel the same pain, you still feel pain – hers and yours for you know it may not end well. You worry, but you must still carry on. Someone has to and it has to be you. There are kids to raise and a job to keep. Insurance, work, school, all of the complexities of life still go on. It was a job I gladly accepted and would do again without hesitation. I was lucky in that I had her mother to help and her friends came by often to help and give me a break. Without them, I truly don't know how I would have gotten through it all. Should you find yourself in this situation, do not hesitate to seek help and guidance. You will need it all, but please remember that you are not alone.

Chapter 29

I Believe In Miracles

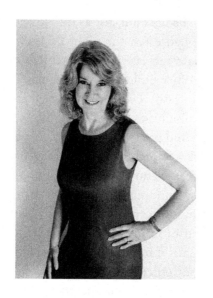

By Sharon Sigler

Do you believe in miracles? Well I do! This is my story of being diagnosed with cancer at the young age of 34! From the start, miracles and angels surrounded me.

It was a rainy, gloomy Monday, October 5, 1992. Like many of my Mondays, I was begrudgingly hurrying out of the house and getting in my car for the long commute to my job in Atlanta. I lived about an hour away from my job in Gwinnett County. My job was located on the other side of I-285, the perimeter in DeKalb County. When I got up that morning, I remember putting my pantyhose on and just hearing this "glut glut glut" sound in my abdominal area. I just figured it was hunger pains. When I got about halfway to my job on I-285 at Ashford Dunwoody Road exit, I got a sharp pain in my abdominal area. I dismissed it just as digestive issues, possibly gas from something I had eaten the night before. As I continued on the highway the pain increased more. I remember praying "just let me make it to my office building." Unfortunately, traffic got in my way and I was sitting still. Eventually I got off my exit and I had to travel another 10 minutes to my office building. I quickly drove up to my office condo and parked. I was feeling very weak to the point that I may faint! I was scared. I had never felt this way before. I took some deep breaths and gathered my strength to get out of the car to head into my building. But after exiting and locking the car door, a wave of faintness came over my body again. I grabbed onto the trunk of my car to steady myself. I was standing outside of my car leaning up against it because I was so weak. ANGEL #1 in my story came out of my office building. He was a delivery person in a brown suit and he came up to me and said" Ma'am are you OK?" I looked at him and said "I don't think I am ok. I feel very weak and I believe I'm going to faint. If I do faint please go to the second floor of this building and ask for Tony. Then apparently I fainted and he caught me. He laid me out on the sidewalk and went upstairs to get my manager Tony. When Tony came outside, I had awoken. He picked me up and carried me into the elevator for the ride upstairs. He insisted on calling 911 and I kept resisting.

Upon exiting the elevator, he put me down and I went into the bathroom thinking I had digestive issues. But after using the restroom, I still felt very weak. I realized that something was truly wrong and I agreed that 911 should be called. I rested painfully in a chair while waiting. The EMT arrived within 5 minutes because Windy Hill Hospital was just down the street. They came in and took my vitals, hoisted me onto the gurney and carried me out to the ambulance. I had never been in an ambulance before. I saw my colleague Bonnie just arriving to work and I said, "Bonnie I don't know what is wrong, I am so scared. Have someone call Larry to come to the hospital." Bonnie said, "Everything will be ok." Years later recollecting this day Bonnie said that I was so white and weak looking, she was so concerned.

Upon arriving at Windy Hill Hospital, I was rushed into a triage room and questions were asked. The main question was "are you pregnant?" They thought it could be an ectopic pregnancy. I told them I was not pregnant. Eventually Larry arrived. I began crying because I was so scared. Larry is my rock and comfort. I just remember being soooo cold and scared in that hospital, I was just shivering. Blood was drawn and tests were taken including an ultrasound test. Apparently this test showed what the problem was. I had a tumor the size of a grapefruit encapsulating my right ovary and it had hemorrhaged. I was losing major amounts of blood internally.

Angel #2 enters the story. His name was Dr. Kenneth Twiddy and he was the gynecologic surgeon on call that Monday morning. Apparently he normally didn't work on Mondays, but was there this particular Monday. Word had it that he was one of the best gynecologic surgeons in the city. He came to talk with me to let me know what was happening and that he would have to perform emergency surgery. I remember he had this soothing voice as he explained the procedure, which helped calm me down immensely. I was to have an epidural that would cause me no feeling from my chest down. For some reason, I was so scared that if they did that, it would affect my breathing and I could die while under sedation. The anesthesiologist assured me that would not happen. When I had to sign the paperwork for permission of the surgery, my hand was shaking so much from fear that my name wasn't legible! I had not been sick in a hospital much less had surgery before.

My parents had come to visit me in the hospital via my husband's urgent phone call. After the surgery, Dr. Twiddy came into the ICU to inform us in his soothing voice, what had happened. He said that it was an ovarian tumor that was cancerous. He believed it was a germ cell yolk-sac type ovarian tumor, but wanted to send it to pathology for diagnosis. He believed he got all the cancer cells removed, but if not, I may have to have another surgery in two weeks.

CANCER???? What? Me? No way!!! I've been healthy, how could I have cancer? I was groggy still from the anesthesia, but I was still able to process this part of the message from Dr. Twiddy. It was so surreal that the day before I was at the Atlanta Falcons game in the new Georgia Dome and today I have a diagnosis of cancer!

I spent a few days in the hospital recovering from the surgery. Because Dr. Twiddy had cut across my lower abdominal area, I had a good number of stitches that kept it all intact. To walk upright or to sneeze or laugh presented pain.

While in the hospital, Dr. Twiddy brought in as a consultant, a gynecologic oncologist surgeon specialist, Dr. Benedict Benigno. Dr. Benigno was tall with a booming, intimidating, deep voice. Apparently he was an expert in this field. Dr. Benigno explained to me about the type of tumor and that the odds of having it was very rare, but very curable with a 95% cure rate especially if I chose to get chemotherapy. I thought to myself, "Heck I want to live a long life so I better get the chemo." The next few days I was in a surreal state as I was deciding what doctor to choose to be my oncologist.

The oncologist on call at Windy Hill Hospital was Dr. Gerald Goldklang. I was considering him to be my oncologist.

Ever since I was rushed in the EMT to the hospital, my story spread to the local Atlanta ad media/sales community. My job title was National Account Executive for a national radio representative firm. Basically, I represented radio stations from all over the country to sell radio commercials on their stations. I worked with radio stations in the Top 10 Radio markets to the Top 50 Radio Markets inclusive of New York City to Augusta Georgia. The Atlanta ad community is an inclusive community, so when one gets hurt, we all band together in care. I was also on the Board of Directors for a local Atlanta Media Club (ABAC) and knew many local radio station dj's and management. I started receiving flowers and plant deliveries from radio associates from all over the country. My room was filled with so many flowers/plants, they were flowing over into the nurse's desk area! I was so overwhelmed with the outpouring of love and concern for me. I actually received cards, letters, and phone calls from people that I didn't even think knew me! I remembered thinking to myself, "They care enough about me to send me a card/gift/letter?" One of my work associates, Mary, mailed me a card every day to stay in touch and give me the latest goings on at the office. To this day, I still have a plastic bin full of the cards, letters and notes from all those people that cared.

While in the hospital recovering, my Aunt Ellen had mailed me a few books to read. One of them was Love, Medicine and Miracles by Dr. Bernie Siegel. The book was his story about being a surgeon. One day he realized that his patients had become numbers, because he had lost touch with the human aspect of his business. He decided he wanted to do something to change it and have a better bedside manner with his patients. He wanted the patient to feel empowered and not at the mercy of the doctor and the medical community. He believed in the Exceptional Patient, and the healing of the self through mind/body connection. With the information in this book, I became empowered instead of frightened of the course that lay ahead. After interviewing a few oncologists, I chose Dr. Goldklang because of his bedside manner. In the meantime, a week or so after my surgery, I had an outpatient procedure for a port to be implanted into my chest for easier access to my veins for chemo application. At the age of 32 I was quite thin at 115 pounds. I had a lot of pains associated with the procedure. When I breathed, my whole chest area hurt. Later that week on Friday, I went to talk with Dr. Goldklang about the upcoming week's chemo schedule. I mentioned to him that I was really hurting and uncomfortable from the procedure. He said, "Let's see how you feel on Monday and we can get an x-ray then. We may have to put off chemo that day." There was a strong voice inside of me that said "No don't wait. You don't want to endure this pain all weekend." Because of my sense of patient empowerment from reading Love, Medicine and Miracles, I said to him, "No I want an x-ray today." The x-ray was performed. I was immediately admitted to the hospital because the x-ray showed I had a collapsed lung. The doctors thought, because I was so thin, my lung may have been nicked when the port was implanted. I was so mad, not necessarily at the Doctor, but the circumstances! Here in the past two weeks, I had endured OC surgery, post-surgery pain and now I have pain from a collapsed lung??

So I was admitted to Windy Hill Hospital. Immediately to relieve my pain, they had to insert a tube in my left side to inflate the lung. They gave me a shot of morphine first to relieve the pain and I am glad they did. That tube insertion was a hell of a pain!!! I was in the hospital for 3 days. I am a pretty even keeled, don't want to be a troublemaker kind of patient. We all know that on weekends, the staff at a hospital is diminished, inclusive of the doctors on call. Each day I would ask to see the doctor, but I did not hear from him. By the third day, I was so ready to leave!! For hours, Hospital staff was telling me they were trying to locate the doctor, but there was no response. Again, because I had read Love, Medicine and Miracles, I felt empowered and basically "threw a fit" to get the doctor to come immediately. Apparently, hospital staff was so taken aback that the doctor appeared within the hour to sign my release papers.

The next day I found out that the pathology report came back that all the cancer had been removed and I did not have to return for a second surgery. I went in that week for my first chemo treatment. Now because I had such a potent set of chemo drugs administered to me, Dr. Goldklang wanted me to be admitted to the hospital for five days straight, one time per month, for the next three months of October, November and December, with daily chemo injections. That meant that I would be in the hospital on Thanksgiving week and the week after Christmas. The reason was that these chemo drugs could have such a devastating effect on my internal organs and they wanted to flush them out with saline solutions immediately afterwards.

I had such high anxiety that first chemo treatment that they had to give me an anti-anxiety drug to calm me down. I mean this is POISON going into my body to kill cancer cells, as well as the good cells too. The "chemo lady" administering the drugs was even dressed in protective garb. After injection, she would say "Now you're cooking with gas." I actually have a photo of her standing over my bed in her protective garb.

The chemo administered into my body took a couple of hours and began in late afternoon. Then for the next several hours into the night the saline solution bags were administered to flush all those nasty poisons/toxins out. I spent hours into the night getting out of bed with my "pole" rolling beside me into the bathroom to pee out all the toxins. Usually by 2AM I was able to settle down for a sleep. Word spread in October that I was getting chemo treatments in the hospital, so I had many friends, family and business acquaintances come by to see me. I am a funny and quick witted person, so when they came by I would joke about my situation with them. I told

243

them "None of this sad stuff, let's be thankful for surviving the surgery because I nearly died from losing all that blood, not from the cancer!" I lost 5 pints of blood!

In 1992, the Atlanta Braves played in the World Series. I was fortunate enough to get two tickets to Game One at Atlanta Fulton County Stadium. (I knew a guy John who was up in ranks at CNN/Turner). I went with my good friend Vickie, who was a Media Buyer at a local ad agency. Braves fever was running rampant across the ATL Metro! It was an exciting time in the city. Vickie and I took a taxi to the stadium from a hotel we had parked at in Buckhead. The taxi was not able to drive us directly up to the stadium front gates and stopped at the edge of the front parking lot. I was still recovering from my original OC surgery, so I didn't have all my strength back yet. Vickie and I walked across the parking lot, on that cool Saturday night. We arrived at the stadium and an usher took us down to our seats, which were in the first few rows behind first base!!! It was an exciting game and Atlanta did end up winning the game against Toronto Blue Jays. Unfortunately, around the seventh inning, I literally ran out of energy. So much so that I knew that I could not walk back up all those steps to get out of the stadium. Vickie was able to flag an usher down and we told him my situation. Upon leaving he put his arm around my waist and helped me up the steps. He was a tall big framed guy, so I could lean on him as we were going up the stairs to diminish the strain on my body. Vickie was following behind us. As we walked up the stairs, fans along the way were watching us because they probably thought I was drunk and was needing assistance to get up the stairs. To this day Vickie and I laugh about this story.

Mind over matter is definitely true when it comes to a catastrophic illness. I had read how the visual the mind sees, has an effect on the body. I decided I would take a red marker and the yearly calendar and put a big X in the box to mark each date I had completed chemo in the hospital. Each Red X represented accomplishment!! I can't tell you how crucial this act of accomplishment was to my overall emotional stamina. In hindsight, I wish I had kept that calendar. It represents to me to this day that I can overcome anything if I put my mind to it. Yes it was the skill and expertise of my doctors to keep me healthy, but it was also my will and determination to live that also played a factor in my survival.

At night in the hospital, after the chemo treatments, I would lay in bed and wonder why this happened to me. Why? I was young. I was nice. I didn't treat people mean. I was always willing to help others and obey the Girl Scout creed (I was a Girl Scout). Why did this happen to me? Why did a bad thing happen to a good person? I would sob out loud asking these questions to God.

It was during these times in the hospital with myself that I began my spiritual inner journey. I had not been brought up with a religion on a consistent basis. My parents growing up were both Christians (Catholic). They never instilled in me and my sisters a ritual of weekly church attendance. Growing up I would attend Sunday school with my Christian friends from time to time. But up to this point in my life, I had not really delved into exploration of God and spirituality. Another one of the books that Aunt Ellen had given me was Seat of the Soul by Gary Zukov. I began reading it in the hospital. It made sense as to my place in the world. Gary talked about authentic power and not succumbing to the feelings of powerlessness. Authentic power is not ego centric power, it is God power. Gary's book embarked me on a journey of finding my inner soul and spirit. Thereafter I read many other well-known, New Age authors from Wayne Dyer to James Redfield to Marianne Williamson and Self Healer Louise Hay to name a few.

It was through these authors that I began to understand the symbiotic relationship between the mind, emotions, body and spirit (MEBS). Throughout these years as an OC survivor, this has been my foundation for staying well. Yes, what we think, thus we become!

245

The 'ol hair falling out story. Well as with most chemo takers, the hair started falling out one day while I was taking a shower. A chunk of hair came out in my hand. It really is a sobering feeling to see that wad of your own hair in your hand. I stood there and cried. I cried because of the powerlessness I had over the situation. Something had invaded my body that I had no control over, CANCER! Then I allowed another something to kill the original something that is wreaking even more havoc in my body! CHEMO! The next day I called my hair stylist Steve and told him what happened. Wonderful Steve came over to my house since I was too weak to leave my house and gave me a fashionable buzz cut.

After that buzz cut, I purchased fashionable turbans in all the popular colors, including red and black turbans for UGA Georgia Bulldawgs colors and a general purpose white one. Then I visited a wig shop that a friend of the family, Ms. Marie owned. I picked out two curly Farrah Fawcett wigs….. one in blond and one brown haired. It really is all about the attitude. Yes I was sad about the hair loss…. however, I told myself that Sharon Gilloolly Sigler is MORE THAN MY HAIR! It was what is on the inside of me, my spirit and my soul that mattered more. Those words became my daily mantra.

In November, I was in the hospital for my chemo treatments on Thanksgiving Day. I had been in the hospital since Monday. The nausea that I felt from the chemo made me not a good candidate for a big Thanksgiving Day meal. Thank goodness Zofran, the anti-nausea drug, had been introduced to the cancer patient in 1992, because it helped me a lot to not ever have to vomit once! I had nausea, but never the need to vomit. Somehow, I felt victorious over this little fact. My dear friend Gary Maigret (R.I.P.) came to visit me on Thanksgiving Day. He brought to me a complete homemade Thanksgiving dinner he had cooked himself for his friends and family. I felt so loved because there were many other places and things to do that Gary could have done, yet he chose to visit me. He had the kindest heart! I told him thank you, but I just could not stomach that food. I did pick at the sweet potatoes though.

December 28-December 31, 1992 were my last four days of chemo treatment! Yahoo! The week after Christmas was not a fun week to go to the hospital for chemo treatments. I had to do everything in my power and God's power to gather the courage to go! But I also knew that this would be my last chemo treatment EVER!!! I brought my calendar with me and put the big RED X through each day I received chemo. Four, three, two and ONE! My last chemo treatment was on the last day of 1992! Happy New Year 1993! I told myself that I was not in remission, that I was cancer free! Thereafter, if a person asked me how long I was in remission, I corrected them and said "My belief system is that I am cancer free and not in remission." I had taken a short- term leave from my work. Mid-January 1993 it was time for me to go back to work. I was looking forward to going back to my job and seeing my colleagues. However, I did not realize the toll working a full eight hour job plus an hour commute each way would have on my stamina. It busted my stamina. I was so fatigued from the effects of the chemo. I would come home each day from work and be so exhausted that I would cry. I feared that the cancer had come back and that is why I was so fatigued. Finally, after a couple of months I told my Manager Tony that I had come back to work too soon and was still too ill to perform my job. He was so understanding and held my job position open longer!

Life as a Cancer Survivor

In April 1993, my Mom and I went to San Francisco, CA for my sisters (twins Maureen and Linda's) 40th birthday party. My hubby, Larry, stayed back here in Atlanta to work. It was a time of family togetherness and love. It was a time also for more recuperation for me. California is such a scenic place with its rising hills and fantastic weather. I took walks in my sister's subdivision, starting off a little at a time to build my stamina up. Those days, I had anxiety as a cancer survivor. Any time I would have an unexplained ache, I would wonder if cancer had come back. While out in California, my sister Linda's husband passed away from cancer. It was a scary time for me because I was a survivor and he was dying.

In May 1993, I went to visit my Aunt Ellen, my Dad's sister, at her home in Nyack, NY. She had a beautiful home stationed along the banks of the Hudson River. It was like staying at a beautiful northern resort! My soul felt restored when I visited her home and gardens. She eats organic healthy nutritional food, which was an introduction to me for a healthier way of eating. Shortly before my stay was over, Ellen invited me to accompany her to the Tony Awards. As a past Tony Award winner for Best Actress for "Same Time Next Year", Aunt Ellen, renowned actress Ellen Burstyn, was invited to be a presenter. I was so excited to go and said a definite "YES"!! It was something to look forward to that was a deviation from my recovery. I called back to my husband in Atlanta and asked him to ship a few of my long dresses. At the Tony's, I had a glorious time being backstage with Ellen and the other Tony winners and presenters. My hair was starting to grow back in. The hairstylist for the show even styled my short do! After The Tony's show, we went to the After Party at a Grand Ballroom. It was all the things one imagines when you are not a celebrity. We sat at the same table as Gregory Hines. I leaned over to Aunt Ellen and whispered how much I loved Mr. Hines dancing and I would love to dance with him. She said "Why don't you ask him?" I said "Oh no, that would be hard for me to do." But something inside of me said, "Why not, go for it, you just beat cancer." So I leaned over to him and asked him to dance and he said, "YES!" He took my hand and guided me onto the dance floor. We began dancing a slow dance. I was in a surreal universe. I had just gone through the biggest test of my life with cancer, overcame it and now I am dancing in the arms of Gregory Hines!! Tears welled up in my eyes. He looked at me and asked if I was ok? I blushed and relayed the story of what I was just thinking. I told him it was such an honor to be dancing with him after all I had gone through with cancer. He stopped dancing, looked into my eyes and said, "No the honor is mine." I just melted! Years later when he passed away from cancer, I remembered this story with tears in my eyes!

My doctor visits to see Dr. Goldklang for my blood counts were every six weeks. The tumor markers and white blood counts were decreasing each visit. For anyone who has had cancer, there is such anticipation and anxiety in the times of "the wait" for the results of the blood tests. As much as I believed in God's presence, the human fearful part of me would take over at times with fear…. Will cancer come back?

Visits to see Dr. Goldklang became every six months and then after reaching the five years cancer free mark, I would have only yearly visits to see him.

The biggest miracle in my life came to me in February 1995. I became pregnant with only one ovary! In November, my daughter Lauren was born. Dr. Goldklang had told me to wait a couple of years after chemo treatments to try to get pregnant to avoid any complications to the fetus from the effects of the chemo. Miracles do happen. My pregnancy was so much fun. I talked to Baby Lauren in utero and played classical music for her. On November 3rd, that night I noticed some slight discomfort. My sister Diane was in town. She began timing my pains. They got to be about 15 minutes apart. I gathered my husband and we made the long trip to Northside Hospital in Atlanta. I had recorded soothing relaxing music for the trip to the hospital. I played that along the way. After about 9 hours of labor, an ultrasound revealed that she had turned and was in the breech position. At 7am, they prepped me for an emergency caesarian. Shortly thereafter, our beautiful Baby Lauren was gifted to us from God above. I've always told her that gold dust was sprinkled upon her when she was born.

I received six weeks off from work for maternity leave. When it was time to return back to work, my job had been eliminated. This ended up being a blessing in disguise because it gave me a max of 18 months to stay with Lauren. Then after, I had to return back to the business world in order for us to have health insurance. I was so excited to spend the first 18 months of Lauren's life full-time with her. The bonding of mother/daughter is a glorious thing!

In early 1996, I read an article in People magazine about the grand opening of the first Gilda's Club in NYC. Named after Gilda Radner, who passed away from ovarian cancer, the mission of Gilda's Club was to provide men, women and children living with cancer a place to go for their emotional and social support. I thought that this would be a wonderful program to have in Atlanta. I called up Joanna Bull, the Executive Director and told her about my story of surviving OC. She sent me a "how to get a chapter started" kit. But upon reading it, I realized with a two month old little baby, I just did not have the time to invest in a startup non-profit. So I put the idea on the back burner for now.

Each year on October 5, I deem it my Celebration of Life day and I take a sabbatical hike to North Georgia to climb either Anna Ruby Falls or Amicalola Falls. It has been my way of showing my gratitude to God for surviving cancer. It is always a glorious time of year because it is Autumn and the leaves are brilliant in their colors. In 1997, I decided to have a Celebration of Life Party, instead of the North Georgia sabbatical. I decided it would be a fundraiser for Gilda's Club and the proceeds would go to the NY Clubhouse. Four hundred dollars was raised. The following year in 1998, I decided to throw a bigger party, raise more money and use it to launch Gilda's Club Greater Atlanta. In my discussion about the event with Gilda's Club NY staff, I was told that another Atlantan was seeking the possibility of bringing a Gilda's Club to Atlanta. Steve Price, an executive at Sears, was organizing a luncheon to raise funds to start a Gilda's Club in Atlanta. Eventually, Steve and I joined forces to establish Gilda's Club Greater Atlanta, a 501-c-3 IRS non-profit organization with approved status in 1998.

Bringing the concept of the Gilda's Club model to Atlanta was important to me because when I had cancer there was no emotional or social support community. Yes I had family and friends to support me, but I never had anyone who I could share my experience with that was going through the same trials and tribulations. Heck, I didn't even know one person who had ovarian cancer. Today in Atlanta, most of the hospitals have their own cancer support programs. However, back then, the Gilda's Club model was one of only two programs that recognized the needs of emotional and social support for cancer patients.

A Board of Directors of Gilda's Club was formed, which I was a member. Because of my connections and relationships in the Atlanta ad/media community, I was able to bring awareness of Gilda's Club to the Atlanta community through radio and TV interviews and various corporate fundraisers and foundation contributions including: The Atlanta Braves Foundation, Powertel, Australian Body Works, Borders Books, the Christmas Homes Tour through Atlanta Homes and Lifestyle Magazine. We also had a Gilda's Club Annual Golf Tournament and the annual Gilda's Club Laugh Off at the Punchline. Eventually Gilda's Club joined with The Wellness Community of Atlanta. Today they are located close to St Joseph and Northside Hospitals as the Cancer Support Community. Recently I visited CSC for the first time. There on the wall was a plaque with the Gilda's Club logo which was the character of Gilda as Rosanna, Rosanna Danna. Tears welled up in my eyes as I realized that my vision of a Gilda's Club had come to fruition!

Another Miracle Story

Back in 2008 around Christmas time, I had a colonoscopy procedure. The results came back questionable, so my gastroenterologist sent the biopsy to the Mayo Clinic for a second opinion. I was anxious about these results, to say the least. I decided to have a virtual group prayer, so I emailed my friends/family/ business colleagues to say a prayer for me on an upcoming date at 6pm. At 6pm that day, I was standing in line at Boston Market ordering food for that night's dinner. I paused to say a prayer for negative results. When I got home and entered my master bathroom, I looked in the mirror and this unbelievable calm fell upon me. A voice came to me, which I considered the voice of God, that said "All is well." This was such a profound moment that I began to cry! The next day was Christmas Eve. I was driving on Hwy I-285 on my way home from work when the call came through from my Doctor with the results. I was nervous as I pushed the green call button. Glory to God the results from Mayo Clinic showed negative for signs of cancer.

My Thank Yous

I wanted to take a few words to give gratitude to my family of yesterday and today. Thank you to my husband Larry. The words of our marriage vows "in sickness and in health" could not be more evident than in the care and devotion that he gave me while I was sick. Larry was a traveling businessman and kept up with the house and our dog those weeks I was either in the hospital or at home recuperating from the surgery or the chemo. To this day he continues to be my rock!

Thank you to my parents Jack and Kitty Gillooly. My parents have always been there to support me, but never to hover or be intrusive in my life. My Dad is now passed away from Alzheimer's disease, but he was a man that was devoted to his family. He was one of the best joke tellers on this planet. I believe he is where I got my silly sense of humor from. My Mom is truly a woman of courage. Born in Czechoslovakia, she endured the loss of her Jewish Father in Auschwitz. After the war, she and her Mom were put in a work camp run by the Russians. She endured terrible living conditions with very limited food to eat. To this day, Mom never throws food away. She says, "when you have been hungry, you never throw food away." In the 60s she had an operation for ulcerative colitis. An infection occurred and she nearly died! My Mom is 85 today and her steady, internal strength keeps her going, despite her profound sadness in losing her only true love, my Dad.

I have three of the most amazing sisters. They don't live in Atlanta anymore, so I only get to see them about once a year. They were born in Germany, whereas I was the only daughter born in the United States We grew up in the Atlanta area in the 50s thru the 70s. When I was sick with cancer, my sisters came to visit me. Thank you to Diane, Linda and Maureen for your sisterly love. As time goes by, we have become even closer in our sisterhood. Thankful for the technology of FaceTime, Skype and texting to keep us connected through the miles. And thank you to our friend Kathy, who is like a sister to me because she lived at our house practically all the time while growing up.

Thank you to my Aunt Ellen (Burstyn). During a very trying period of my life, she was there for me for support. After my cancer diagnosis, she provided books and anecdotal stories of her path of her inner spiritual journey. I read her book, "Lessons in Becoming Myself", which gave me great insight of the great stamina she has in order to survive in the acting industry.

Thank you to members in the medical community for saving my life that rainy October day and keeping me health in the ensuing years since: Thank you to Dr. Kenneth Twiddy, Dr. Benedict Benigno, Dr. Gerald Goldklang, Dr. Catherine Bonk and Dr. Ito (RIP), and Dr. Ravikanth.

Thank you to my nephew Brett Butler. He has grown up to be a handsome man with the funniest personality. I tell him he still has not missed his chance to be a stand up comedian.

Finally, thank you to my wonderful daughter, Lauren. She truly is a miracle gift from God. Growing up, I knew she was an old soul, because of the profound things that emanated from her mouth. Sometimes I would look at her and say, "Now how old are you because what you just said, a four year old would not know to ask that!" She is that grounded person that I wanted to aspire to be when I was her age. I have so enjoyed watching her bloom into the soon to be 21 year old that she has become.

Lauren and Sharon's Favorite Song:
I Hope You Dance by LeAnn Womack

I hope you never lose your sense of wonder,
You get your fill to eat but always keep that hunger,
May you never take one single breath for granted,
GOD forbid love ever leave you empty handed,
I hope you still feel small when you stand beside the ocean,
Whenever one door closes I hope one more opens,
Promise me that you'll give faith a fighting chance,
And when you get the choice to sit it out or dance.
I hope you dance....I hope you dance.
I hope you never fear those mountains in the distance,
Never settle for the path of least resistance
Livin' might mean takin' chances but they're worth takin',
Lovin' might be a mistake but it's worth makin',
Don't let some hell bent heart leave you bitter,
When you come close to sellin' out reconsider,
Give the heavens above more than just a passing glance,
And when you get the choice to sit it out or dance. I hope you dance....I hope you dance.
I hope you dance....I hope you dance.
(Time is a wheel in constant motion always rolling us along,
Tell me who wants to look back on their years and wonder where those years have gone.)

Twenty-four Years of Success

Many people ask me how I am able to be a long term survivor of such a deadly disease, of ovarian cancer. Below are practices that I have incorporated into my daily life:

- The type of ovarian cancer I had was NOT the "garden variety" that many women are diagnosed with. Mine was rarer and more curable.
- With chemo, survivorship increases into the 90% ranking.
- I practice the combination of self-healing including mind, emotions, body, and spirit (MEBS).
- I journal my emotions. When I am filled with various emotions that are hard to sort through, I journal those emotions. Evidence based research shows that writing our emotions down releases those emotions from our tense bodies. Our blood pressure decreases.
- I laugh as often as I can. Laughter is the best medicine. Yes the world can be a scary place. However, it is also a place of love and laughter. It all depends on what lens you choose to look at life through.
- Guided imagery or visualization---again evidence based research shows that when you have a visual image of what your goal is, it releases calming chemicals into our bodies. I call it going to my happy place. For me my happy place is the beach. When I was sick, I actually took a sabbatical to the beach. I laid at the water's edge of the Atlantic Ocean and had the water wash over my body. I envisioned the water washing over me and taking the cancer cells away from my body. I took this powerful experience and tucked it away into my being. To this day it is this image of the feel of the sun, and sand and the sound of the ocean waves that relaxes me when I get in places of anxiety.

- Meditation and diaphragmatic breathing- learning to breathe from our diaphragm is one of the most healing things we can do. It allows the oxygen to go far and wide into our bodies. Meditation calls the mind, which calms the body.
- Nutritious foods- I have learned to eat the "right" foods most of the time. My digestive tract seems to be sensitive, so I learned to limit my intake of dairy, spicy foods and beef products. Now that I am in my 50s, I am also limiting sugar, simple carbs, no artificial sweeteners, chocolate and coffee. I eat more proteins and plant based foods. I drink half my height of 65 inches in 32 ounces of water daily.
- Exercise- the benefits of exercising our bodies is enormous, especially as a cancer survivor. Throughout most of my life, I was blessed to basically not have to always watch what I eat or exercise because God blessed me with good genes for slenderness. However, evidence based research shows the healing effects of exercise from lowering blood pressure, lowering cholesterol, keeping fat ratio in check, releasing positive endorphins into our bodies that keep us happy and upbeat and help us to sleep better. I don't like it but I do it to stay healthy.
- Sleep-New evidence based research shows that deep REM sleep has a healing effect on our brains and bodies. Eight hours minimum of nightly sleep restores the circuits in our brain. Back 24 years ago, we didn't have the technology of personal phones, I-pads, etc., we have now that can interrupt our sleep cycles.
- Love Makes the World Go Round- I choose to have love in my heart vs. anger and resentment. It creates harmony in our bodies vs disharmony in our bodies.
- Believe in Myself - Before cancer, I really looked at other people's lives and wanted to be like them. Many seemed

to have a charmed life. However, I have learned that things are not what they appear to be.

- Acceptance- this is a big word. I spent many years trying to change myself and even others for what my perception of what I wanted them/ me to be. I discovered that "keeping up with the Jones" was just a perception that was not benefiting me. What and who says we have to look outward to compare ourselves to others ...Because society says so? I rose above it and I put that energy into more substantial endeavors like volunteering my time to help others

- Letting Go-Through the years, due to age and wisdom, I have learned to just let go of things that don't really serve me... Inclusive of feelings and even "stuff" and" things". I am a romantic and sentimentalist, so I like to keep my memories in many boxes in my basement. Now I am learning to take a picture of it and toss the real items! De-cluttering has brought me new energies!

- Spirituality- I believe that there is a God/energy force larger than we are. We are made in the likeness of God, so God is within each of us. When I pray to God, I am praying to God inside of me.

- Balance- it is so easy to get overwhelmed with life. I wore so many different hats in my younger years from wife, Mother, employee, civic obligations, after hours business events, exerciser and church participant. I squeezed way too much time out of those 24 hours! However, on looking back it has been exciting, full years of living with gusto and fun.

- Don't Let the Turkeys Get You Down- when I was younger especially in my business affairs, I would get disappointed in my expectations and outcome of a situation or person. My husband Larry would jokingly quote "don't let the turkeys get you down." I learned to not live with expectations because I can only control myself and I cannot control the actions of other people.

- Listen to my body- when we are young we tend to think we are invincible and we don't listen to our bodies. Before I was rushed to the hospital with the bleeding ovarian tumor, I did have symptoms of ovarian cancer, but I only thought they were part of the life I was living. I was very fatigued, but only assumed it was because of the fast paced life of a radio sales account executive. I had a bloaty abdomen from time to time, but I brushed it off as just digestive issues.
- Gratitude-God's hand was on my life that October 5th day. Because if the tumor had not hemorrhaged, I would not have known it was in my body until a stage 3 or 4 diagnosis. I give thanks to God. I practice daily gratitude for the people in my life, and the place I am in my life.
- Music and dance- music and dance is such a healer to my soul. They bring such joy to me. When I am stressed, I put on my favorite artists and dance. Madonna and I are the same age. Her music has helped me get through trying times. After completing chemo treatments, Gloria Estefan's "Coming Out of the Dark" song spoke to my triumphant feat!
- Having a pet- In my marriage we had 3 cats and one dog all at one time. Eventually they all passed on over the rainbow. Recently, my 12 year old dog passed away suddenly from bloat. She knew me like an old friend. I am still in mourning. She gave me such unconditional love. She was a constant to come home to and now it is a quieter house without her.
- Friendships- As an extrovert, friendships are nourishment to my soul. Throughout my life, I have had many acquaintances and friends. Through the power of Facebook, I have gotten back in touch with childhood friends from my days living in DeKalb County Ga,

my high school friends in Cobb County, GA and my Kappa Delta sisters from the University of Georgia. Shout outs to childhood neighbor Cheryl Garman Neill, Lisa Sarajian, Cindy Peters Knoess; business colleagues Judy Maloney, Cathi Johansen, Robyn Sawczyn, and Vickie Martin; Snellville GA neighbor Leisa Violette, KD Sisters roommates; Kathleen Bradshaw, Pam Chadwick Steele. Debbie Habuda Brazeal, Cathy Grimland Ottley, Dorothy Dawkins Boyd, April Sams Halliday and Terri Atkinson Candler. KD sisters that always made me laugh, Libba Schell and Norma Hastings and our wonderful leadership of DeDe Parsons Guest.

- Talk Psychotherapy- Cognitive based talk psychotherapy really has helped me sort through problem times in my life… for example living through cancer. It changes the circuitry of the brain for the better and keeps anxiety in check.

- Famous Quotes- They nourish my soul. I use them as guides for my life. Marianne Williamson, Martin Luther King and Joseph Campbell have powerful messages for me.

- "Our deepest fear is not that we are inadequate. Our deepest fear is that we are powerful beyond measure. It is our light, not our darkness that most frightens us. We ask ourselves, 'Who am I to be brilliant, gorgeous, talented, fabulous?' Actually, who are you not to be? You are a child of God. Your playing small does not serve the world. There is nothing enlightened about shrinking so that other people won't feel insecure around you. We are all meant to shine, as children do. We were born to make manifest the glory of God that is within us. It's not just in some of us; it's in everyone. And as we let our own light shine, we unconsciously give other people permission to do the same. As we are liberated from our

own fear, our presence automatically liberates others."
Marianne Williamson
- "Darkness cannot drive out darkness; only light can do that. Hate cannot drive out hate; only love can do that." Martin Luther King.

- "We must be willing to get rid of
  the life we've planned, so as to have
  the life that is waiting for us.
  The old skin has to be shed
  before the new one can come." Joseph Campbell.

- And the most important quote is from Sharon Sigler:
- "A good hearty laugh daily is good for your soul!!

Ecclesiastes 3:1
To everything there is a season
And a time to every purpose under the Heaven
A time to be born, and a time to die;
A time to plant and a time to pluck up that which is planted;
A time to kill, and a time to heal;
A time to break down, and a time to build up;
A time to weep, and a time to laugh;
A time to mourn, and a time to dance!

Chapter 30

Blank Stares, Salt Shakers, Robots and a Better Me

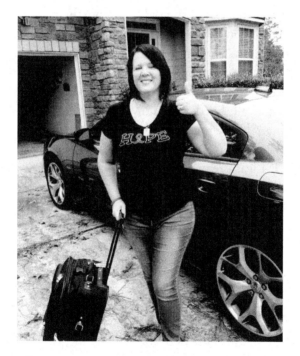

By Kristy Smith

In January 2015 I had a routine appointment with my OB/GYN and mentioned to him that my husband and I had been trying to conceive. I use to say I did not want kids, but seeing how great my husband is with my step-son had me thinking about it more and more. We have been married since 2007. I got off of the pill in 2011 and decided to "just see what happens". So, I mentioned it to my Doctor that day because I had just turned 39 and thought I might be close to starting menopause. I lost my right fallopian tube many years ago and my Doctor suggested checking the other one for blockage. On my way out I talked with the receptionist about scheduling the procedure to check my tube. She said she would give me a call to set up a date and time.

Three months later, I still had not heard from them about scheduling the laparoscopic procedure. I never followed up with them and was back to my "If it's meant to be it will be" mind frame. In mid-April, I kept telling myself I needed to get it scheduled, but days went by and I still hadn't called them. As crazy as it sounds, my dog made me call. She kept following me around and leaning on me, whining. She even pushed her nose into my belly a few times. I would talk to her and say, "Why are you being so needy lately?" I wondered if I was pregnant.

When I did call, I was told that they had tried to call me and had left me messages. It turns out they had one digit of my phone number wrong. So, we scheduled the laparoscopy for a few days later, Tuesday, April 21, 2015. While I was in recovery that day, the Doctor told my husband and mother that the tube looked fine. He also nonchalantly mentioned that he'd seen a few spots/nodules that he took biopsies of but did not think they were anything to worry about. So, the next step would be for me to get on a medicine called Clomid to try to help me get pregnant. I was scheduled to come to his office in 2 weeks to have my stitches removed and get my Clomid prescription. Three days later (Friday) I got a call asking me to come in Tuesday the 28th instead of the following

Tuesday as planned. I was told they were just rearranging some appointments. I didn't think anything of it.

Tuesday, April 28, 2015 I arrived – alone – at the Doctors office. We had a vacation planned for a couple weeks later and I was supposed to be ovulating then, so I was ready to get on the Clomid and go to NYC and get pregnant. While Doc was taking my stitches out I was obviously nervous and I said, "Can you imagine how much of a big baby I am going to be when I am pregnant?" His whole face changed. He pulled up a chair right in front of me, took the pictures from the laparoscopy out of a folder and started explaining them to me.

"This is your ovary, this is the tube… everything here looks good… These spots here, this is what I was a little concerned about. I took a biopsy here, here, here."
Pause ---------------- Blank stare.
"Unfortunately --- the results came back that ---"
Pause -------------- Blank stare.
"There is no easy way to say this, Kristy. It's cancer."

The magnitude of what he said and the turn my life was about to take really did not register in my brain. I was thinking "Ok, they'll just go in and take it out."

"You have ovarian cancer. It has spread from the ovary. You are going to have to have a complete hysterectomy."

That is when it really hit me and the tears and hyperventilating started. I was alone, heartbroken, and terrified. My husband was at work. My Mom had just returned home from a trip to Tennessee. I had no idea how to tell her what I had just heard, or if she would even be able to understand me through the crying. I asked the

Doctor to call her. I don't remember what he said except telling her how to get to his office. He handed me my phone back and she was crying and said, "I'll be right there, ok? I'll be right there."

I text my husband back to back, several times within about 20 seconds, hoping he would hear his phone sound off at work and check it. Instead of the usual "Hey baby, call me when you get a chance"…

Call me
Call me
CALL ME

When I answered his call I couldn't even talk. "What's wrong? What's wrong? Babe? Babe? What's wrong?!" All I could do was cry. Then I managed to blurt out, "I'VE GOT CANCER!" I tried to explain what I could but don't really know what I said. I do remember telling him there was no need in him getting off work early because he'd be off in a couple hours anyway. He ignored that, of course.

The same thing pretty much happened with my best friend. "Where are you? I'll be right there." I just sat there, numb, trying to control my breathing, wondering if I was about to die.

I had a CT scan three days later. It did not show any tumors outside of my abdomen. That was a huge relief! I met with an Oncologist a couple days after that and he told me that judging from the pictures that were taken during the laparoscopic procedure, it looked like someone had taken a salt shaker and sprinkled cancer all over my abdomen. Believe me when I tell you, I have not looked at a salt shaker the same since then.

I had my hysterectomy and debulking surgery on May 28, 2015. It was exactly one month since my diagnosis. It's amazing how fast life can change. The oncologist told me that he was going to remove my omentum. I had never heard of that and it freaked me out and made me wonder if they would have to take anything else out once they could see everything.

Surgery went well. The cancer had indeed spread through my entire abdomen. We didn't know how badly until the surgery. Other than my reproductive organs, it attacked my pelvic tissue, bottom of my stomach, upper abdominal lining and diaphragm. I constantly wondered how long I'd had cancer and not known it. I still wonder about that.

Being surgically thrown into menopause was no fun at all! (An Understatement!) On top of that, I had to start taking anti-estrogen meds because my cancer was fed by estrogen. (ER+) The hot flashes were unbearable. I felt like a stranger in my own body. I stood in the mirror many times and just stared at my scar. Sometimes I would think that if it was horizontal like a C-section scar it would be easier to hide from myself. But of course, it is a long vertical scar. One day I said it looked like someone tried to cut me in half. Right then, I realized that I should be proud of the scar. Cancer tried to kill me and I am still here. That became my motto. I AM STILL HERE.

I don't know if I had much of the emotional effects of menopause because I was already on such an emotional roller coaster. I have such a great support system that really helped me in ways I could never explain or repay. My family and close friends really supported me during this tough time! There were plenty of times I felt scared, defeated and worried, but they made me feel inspired, determined and powerful. Even strangers reached out to me. I was blown away by all of the support and encouragement. I heard from people that I never thought would reach out to me. Old friends, former co-workers, even my favorite football team helped me keep fighting on days that I really did not want to. My husband and I are huge

Atlanta Falcons fans. Their organization and fan base supported me through my battle and still inspire me today. Everyone that visited, brought meals, called, sent cards, etc., will always hold a special place in my heart. I never realized how important things like that were. Now that I can understand it because of the impact it had on me, I am determined to pay it forward.

On my 40th birthday, November 10, 2015, I was told that I needed a second surgery and chemotherapy. I started wondering if it was going to be an on-going thing. I was depressed and afraid. More importantly, I got angry. My anger actually helped me fight. I would get mad enough that I would do what I needed or wanted to do in spite of how I was feeling.

I had a "Second Look Surgery" on December 1, 2015 and started chemo 2 weeks later. I remember one afternoon a few days after my first chemo treatment, I wanted so badly to take a shower but was very weak and in pain. I could hardly stand. I wasn't allowed to take a bath yet because I had to wait 3 weeks after surgery. I had one more week to go. I thought about doing it anyway but didn't want to risk anything by going against Doctors orders. I just laid in bed and cried and cried. Then, I got pissed. I got up, stumbled to the shower and literally talked to cancer the whole time I was bathing. I cursed at it, I yelled at it, I told it that it was not going to define me or control me. My husband helped me get out of the shower and back in bed. I was so exhausted but I felt victorious.

Chemo was strange. It felt like an out of body experience – sitting there watching poison go in to my body. I felt yucky sometimes and had bouts of "chemo brain" but mostly I was just tired, sore, and weak. Overall, with the help of my nausea meds, I tolerated chemo pretty well. The only exception was after my third chemo; I got horribly sick and was hospitalized for 6 days. I have never felt so bad in my life. I talked to God and told him "If this is how I am going to die, please, just take me now. I can't do this anymore."

I told my Mom and my husband "I'm over it. I'm not doing this anymore." To this day I feel really bad for saying that even though I totally meant it at the time. I know it worried them and I feel guilty about that.

We thought the chemo had (directly) made me sick but it turns out an infection had gotten into my bloodstream because my immune system was weakened from the chemo. So, at my next appointment, my Doctor gave me Neulasta to boost my white blood cell counts and keep my immune system in check. It is a small box that attaches to the arm and has medicine in it that injects into your body the day after chemo. It feels like an electric shock. I felt like a robot wearing that thing on my arm but was amazed by it. My last 3 chemo treatments went well.

On February 22, 2016 I had my fourth chemotherapy treatment. When I saw my Doctor he told me that I was in remission. REMISSION! Music to my ears! I did it! I made it! Its official! I did a "happy dance" and was so excited about making phone calls to spread the good news. I made a couple of calls in the waiting area. My husband suggested waiting until I got in to my private room for chemo before making more calls. It was a solemn reminder that not everyone around me was celebrating good news. His reminder was based on the fact that the day we left the Doctors office after learning I had cancer, there was a very happy and excited woman in the parking lot on the phone saying, "She's having a girl! It's a girl! It's a girl!" which made me even more upset that day

.

On April 4, 2016, while being cheered on by my nurses, my husband, Mom, dad, brother, best friend, step son & step Mom, I rang the bell to celebrate my last chemo. On the bell it says, "There comes a point in almost everyone's life when your world is turned upside down, and you know immediately that life as you knew it is forever changed... you realize that from that Moment on, your life will be divided into two parts... before this and after this. –

Author Unknown". I have definitely thought of things in my life as "before cancer…" and "after my diagnosis…"

Looking back, I am just so thankful that the cancer was found when it was. I am so glad that I made that phone call and scheduled the procedure that allowed the Doctor to see the cancer. I'll never forget that Doctor telling me, "trying to bring a life into this world saved your life." So many women are not diagnosed until Stage 4 when the disease has spread outside of the abdomen and the survival rate plummets. I was knocking on Stage Four's door. I had the symptoms of ovarian cancer but never knew what they were. I do not understand why it is not talked about more, especially at Doctors' offices and especially because there is no reliable screening for it.

Looking ahead, honestly, I am afraid it will come back. But I am also thankful for the chance to do things I have always wanted to do, and spend more time on what matters in life. I know I am a better person now. A better wife, daughter, sister, mother, friend, employee… every part of my life has been touched by cancer.

It did not destroy me and I will not let my survival be in vain. I do wonder about recurrence, but I do not dwell on it. I'd much rather concentrate on making the best out of every day that I am given. Whatever may come my way, I know that I have lived a good life and been a good person. I am at peace with whatever God has planned for me.

If you'd like to see more about my fight and what encourages me, please check out my YouTube videos; "How Football Inspires Me" and "My Final Words for Cancer" .

CPSIA information can be obtained
at www.ICGtesting.com
Printed in the USA
FSOW03n1232310117
30094FS